Endocrinology

Editor

JI HYUN CHUN (CJ)

PHYSICIAN ASSISTANT CLINICS

www.physicianassistant.theclinics.com

Consulting Editor
JAMES A. VAN RHEE

January 2017 • Volume 2 • Number 1

ELSEVIER

1600 John F. Kennedy Boulevard • Suite 1800 • Philadelphia, Pennsylvania, 19103-2899

http://www.theclinics.com

PHYSICIAN ASSISTANT CLINICS Volume 2, Number 1
January 2017 ISSN 2405-7991, ISBN-13: 978-0-323-48267-7

Editor: Jessica McCool
Developmental Editor: Casey Potter

Physician Assistant Clinics (ISSN: 2405–7991) is published quarterly by Elsevier Inc., 360 Park Avenue South, New York, NY 10010-1710. Months of issue are January, April, July, and October. Periodicals postage paid at New York, NY and additional mailing offices. Subscription prices are $150.00 per year (US individuals), $205.00 (US institutions), $100.00 (US students), $210.00 (Canadian individuals), $257.00 (Canadian institutions), $100.00 (Canadian students), $150.00 (international individuals), $257.00 (international institutions), and $100.00 (international students). Foreign air speed delivery is included in all *Clinics* subscription prices. All prices are subject to change without notice. POSTMASTER: Send address changes to *Physician Assistant Clinics*, Elsevier Periodicals Customer Service, 11830 Westline Industrial Drive, St. Louis, MO 63146. Customer Service Health Sciences Division, Subscription Customer Service, 3251 Riverport Lane, Maryland Heights, MO 63043. **Customer Service: 1-800-654-2452 (U.S. and Canada); 314-447-8871 (outside U.S. and Canada). Fax: 314-447-8029. E-mail: journalscustomerservice-usa@elsevier.com (for print support); journalsonlinesupport-usa@elsevier.com (for online support).**

Reprints. For copies of 100 or more, of articles in this publication, please contact the Commercial Reprints Department, Elsevier Inc., 360 Park Avenue South, New York, NY 10010-1710. Tel. 212-633-3874; Fax: 212-633-3820; E-mail: reprints@elsevier.com.

Physician Assistant Clinics is covered in *MEDLINE/PubMed (Index Medicus)* and *EMBASE/Excerpta Medica, Current Contents/Clinical Medicine,* and *ISI/BIOMED.*

PROGRAM OBJECTIVE
The goal of the Physician Assistant Clinics is to keep practicing physician assistants up to date with current clinical practice by providing timely articles reviewing the state of the art in patient care.

TARGET AUDIENCE
Physician Assistants and other healthcare professionals.

LEARNING OBJECTIVES
Upon completion of this activity, participants will be able to:
1. Review standards of care in the treatment of common endocrine disorders.
2. Discuss the evaluation, workup, and treatment of thyroid and parathyroid disorders.
3. Recognize treatment standards and special considerations for conditions such as diabetes mellitus, obesity, and adrenal disorders, among others.

ACCREDITATION
The Elsevier Office of Continuing Medical Education (EOCME) is accredited by the Accreditation Council for Continuing Medical Education (ACCME) to provide continuing medical education for physicians.

The EOCME designates this enduring material for a maximum of 15 *AMA PRA Category 1 Credit*(s)™. Physicians should claim only the credit commensurate with the extent of their participation in the activity.

All other health care professionals requesting continuing education credit for this enduring material will be issued a certificate of participation.

DISCLOSURE OF CONFLICTS OF INTEREST
The EOCME assesses conflict of interest with its instructors, faculty, planners, and other individuals who are in a position to control the content of CME activities. All relevant conflicts of interest that are identified are thoroughly vetted by EOCME for fair balance, scientific objectivity, and patient care recommendations. EOCME is committed to providing its learners with CME activities that promote improvements or quality in healthcare and not a specific proprietary business or a commercial interest.

The planning committee, staff, authors and editors listed below have identified no financial relationships or relationships to products or devices they or their spouse/life partner have with commercial interest related to the content of this CME activity:
Sonia L. Bahroo, PA-C; Karen Beer, PA-C, MSPAS, RD, LD, CDE; Joseph Daniel; Joy A. Dugan, MPH, MSPAS, PA-C; Anjali Fortna; Casey Jackson; Jessica McCool; Shannon McShea, PA-C, MSPAS, CNSC; Melissa Murfin, PA-C, PharmD, BCACP; Sondra O'Callaghan, PA-C, MPH, CHES; Sheila Pinkson, MPAS, BS, PA-C; Kristen A. Scheckel, PA-C; Ashlyn Smith, MMS, PA-C; Megan Suermann.

The planning committee, staff, authors and editors listed below have identified financial relationships or relationships to products or devices they or their spouse/life partner have with commercial interest related to the content of this CME activity:
Ji Hyun Chun (CJ), MPAS, PA-C, BC-ADM is on the speakers' bureau for AbbVie Inc, and is a consultant/advisor for GSK group of companies; AstraZeneca; Sanofi; Shire; Takeda Pharmaceuticals U.S.A., Inc.
James Van Rhee, MS, PA-C receives royalties/patents from Kaplan, Inc.
Christopher Sadler, MA, PA-C, CDE has stock ownership in, and has an employment affiliation with, AstraZeneca.

UNAPPROVED/OFF-LABEL USE DISCLOSURE
The EOCME requires CME faculty to disclose to the participants:
1. When products or procedures being discussed are off-label, unlabelled, experimental, and/or investigational (not US Food and Drug Administration [FDA] approved); and
2. Any limitations on the information presented, such as data that are preliminary or that represent ongoing research, interim analyses, and/or unsupported opinions. Faculty may discuss information about pharmaceutical agents that is outside of FDA-approved labelling. This information is intended solely for CME and is not intended to promote off-label use of these medications. If you have any questions, contact the medical affairs department of the manufacturer for the most recent prescribing information.

TO ENROLL
The CME program is available to all Physician Assistant Clinics subscribers at no additional fee. To subscribe to the Physician Assistant Clinics, call customer service at 1-800-654-2452 or sign up online at www.physicianassistant.theclinics.com.

METHOD OF PARTICIPATION

In order to claim credit, participants must complete the following:
1. Complete enrolment as indicated above.
2. Read the activity.
3. Complete the CME Test and Evaluation. Participants must achieve a score of 70% on the test. All CME Tests and Evaluations must be completed online.

CME INQUIRIES/SPECIAL NEEDS

For all CME inquiries or special needs, please contact elsevierCME@elsevier.com.

Contributors

CONSULTING EDITOR

JAMES VAN RHEE, MS, PA-C
Associate Professor, Program Director, Yale University, Yale Physician Assistant Program, New Haven, Connecticut

EDITOR

JI HYUN CHUN (CJ), MPAS, PA-C, BC-ADM
President Elect, American Society of Endocrine Physician Assistants; Endocrine Physician Assistant, OptumCare Medical Group, Laguna Niguel, California; Adjunct Faculty, A.T. Still University, Mesa, Arizona

AUTHORS

SONIA L. BAHROO, PA-C
Physician Assistant, Division of Endocrinology, Physician Assistant, Department of Medicine, The George Washington University Medical Faculty Associates, Inc., Washington, DC

KAREN BEER, PA-C, MSPAS, RD, LD, CDE
Physician Assistant, Oregon Medical Group, Eugene, Oregon

JOY A. DUGAN, MPH, MSPAS, PA-C
Adjunct Assistant Professor, Joint MSPAS/MPH Program, Touro University California, Mare Island, California

SHANNON McSHEA, PA-C, MSPAS, CNSC
Physician Assistant, Department of Nutrition and Weight Management, Geisinger Medical Center, Danville, Pennsylvania

MELISSA MURFIN, PA-C, PharmD, BCACP
Academic Coordinator; Assistant Professor, Department of Physician Assistant Studies, Elon University, Elon, North California

SONDRA O'CALLAGHAN, PA-C, MPH, CHES
Division of Endocrinology, NF/SG Veterans Health System, Gainesville, Florida

SHEILA PINKSON, MPAS, BS, PA-C
Adjunct Assistant Professor, Endocrine, University of Texas Health Science Center at San Antonio, San Antonio, Texas; Endocrine Physician Assistant, South Texas Veterans Health Care System, San Antonio, Texas

CHRISTOPHER SADLER, MA, PA-C, CDE
Diabetes and Endocrine Associates, La Jolla, California; AstraZeneca Pharmaceuticals LP, Medical Affairs Department, Wilmington, Delaware

KRISTEN A. SCHECKEL, PA-C
Creekside Endocrine Associates, Denver, Colorado

ASHLYN SMITH, MMS, PA-C
Chief Delegate, American Society of Endocrine Physician Assistants; Current Practicing Physician Assistant, Endocrinology Associates, Scottsdale, Arizona

Contents

Phenotypically people with diabetes do not always match their genotype. Discerning the cause of an individual's diabetes affords an opportunity for optimization of treatment, reduction of complications, and ultimately, amelioration of disease burden.

This article discusses the American Association of Clinical Endocrinologist/ American College of Endocrinologists and American Diabetes Association 2016 guidelines for managing diabetes mellitus types 1 and 2. Although these guidelines exist, patients must also have individualized targets based on age, activity, and comorbidity status. Furthermore, glucose control does not equate to diabetes control, because there are multiple other process and outcome measures, including blood pressure, lipid, and weight control, that contribute to diabetes management. For all patients with diabetes, lifestyle optimization is key.

Selecting the most appropriate medication for patients with diabetes can be daunting, given the ever-expanding list of available medications. Expert guidance comes from the American Diabetes Association *Standards of Medical Care* and the American Association of Clinical Endocrinologists type 2 algorithm. Metformin, diet, and exercise are the recommended initial treatments of patients with newly diagnosed type 2 diabetes mellitus.

Optimizing diabetes treatment is complex, but particularly in patients with special considerations. Elderly patients have numerous, competing issues; pediatric patients have few medications that have been studied in younger people. Minimizing hypoglycemia has come to greater attention with diabetes guideline updates. More attention is also being paid to medications that could be problematic in patients with kidney disease. Polypharmacy is a concern for all patients. With careful attention to prescribing and medication review to identify and prevent problems, providers can manage patients with special considerations, helping them achieve goals and prevent adverse outcomes owing to drug interactions and side effects.

Levothyroxine is the gold standard treatment for hypothyroidism. The use liothyronine is controversial and a constant topic of discussion. It is not advised for routine clinical use of as monotherapy, but can be a good choice for specific subpopulations. Extended or sustained release preparations of liothyronine have been used in research settings with favorable results but because there are no formal pharmacokinetic studies, it is not approved by the US Food and Drug Administration and only available at compounding pharmacies. This opens the door for further clinical trials as well as future development of an extended release liothyronine product.

Serum thyroid-stimulating hormone (TSH) is the appropriate screening test for thyroid dysfunction. A TSH level within the normal range excludes primary thyroid disease. Causes of low TSH are numerous and include Graves disease, toxic multinodular goiter, toxic adenoma, thyroiditis, subclinical hyperthyroidism, medications, pregnancy, secondary hypothyroidism, overtreatment of hypothyroidism, factitious thyroid hormone ingestion, and nonthyroidal illness. Signs and symptoms of thyrotoxicosis include heat intolerance, palpitations, anxiety, fatigue, weight loss, irregular menses in women, tremor, tachycardia, and warm, moist skin. Graves disease is the most common cause of hyperthyroidism. Treatment options include antithyroid drugs, radioactive iodine ablation, and surgery.

Thyroid nodules are commonly encountered in clinical practice during both routine examinations and imaging procedures. Although most thyroid nodules are benign, there is an increasing prevalence of well-differentiated thyroid cancers. Nodules that are suspected to be overactive are best evaluated by laboratory testing to assess thyroid function, radionuclide examination, or thyroid ultrasound (US) examination, which is the preferred imaging procedure. US characteristics can help to identify potentially malignant nodules based on the presence of high-risk US characteristics. Nodules that are determined to be at higher risk for malignancy based on US characteristics are recommended for fine needle aspiration.

Overweight and obesity is an epidemic in the United States affecting more than 60% of the adult population. Obesity and the associated comorbidities greatly affect overall morbidity and mortality. This article reviews the current recommendations from the *2013 AHA/ACC/TOS Guideline for the Management of Overweight and Obesity in Adults,* the available medications for weight loss, and discusses bariatric surgery.

Sheila Pinkson

Pituitary disorders can cause hormonal abnormalities that affect the functions of other glands and neurologic conditions. Rarely are these disorders life threatening. However, there are multiple and sometimes subtle manifestations of these pituitary disorders that can provide a significant challenge in the diagnoses and management of many pituitary conditions. The importance is for early recognition of signs and symptoms of hypersecretion, hyposecretion, and/or mass effects. A multidisciplinary approach should be coordinated with an endocrinologist and other specialties to provide management and follow-up for the best treatment practices.

Kristen A. Scheckel

Although rare, adrenal disorders have always enticed students and practitioners alike. Adrenal disorders should be considered in the differential diagnosis for many clinical presentations. Because most adrenal conditions have potentially life-threatening consequences, proper diagnosis and treatment are crucial. These challenging cases require understanding of underlying pathophysiology, a detailed history, comprehensive physical examination, laboratory assessment, and careful interpretation of imaging studies to make the correct diagnosis. This article highlights clinical features, diagnosis, and treatment strategies for congenital adrenal hyperplasia, adrenal insufficiency, Cushing syndrome, primary aldosteronism, and pheochromocytoma.

Ashlyn Smith

Calcium homeostasis is vital for maintaining normal neurologic and musculoskeletal function and health. Multiple conditions can alter serum calcium levels varying from endocrine disorders and medication effects to immobility, malignancy, and genetic disorders. Because of the diversity of conditions that can cause variations in serum calcium levels, a focused history and physical examination can help narrow down the differential diagnosis in order to limit a "shotgun" approach to the workup. This review explores the common misconceptions that present in evaluating and treating calcium and parathyroid disorders with a comprehensive discussion on appropriate care.

Endocrinology

PHYSICIAN ASSISTANT CLINICS

RELATED INTEREST

Endocrinology and Metabolism Clinics of North America
December 2016 (Vol. 45, Issue 4)
Diabetes
S. Sethu K. Reddy, *Editor*
Available at: http://www.endo.theclinics.com/

THE CLINICS ARE AVAILABLE ONLINE!
Access your subscription at:
www.theclinics.com

Foreword

Almost 30 Million People

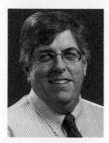

James Van Rhee, MS, PA-C
Consulting Editor

The numbers are staggering: 29.1 million people in the United States have diabetes, 8.1 million of those being undiagnosed. Diabetes is the seventh leading cause of death in the United States. Diabetes is the primary cause of kidney failure in all new cases. Sixty percent of all nontraumatic lower-limb amputations among people over the age of 20 occur in people with diabetes. Cost of diabetes care is $245 billion in the United States.[1] As I said, these numbers are staggering, but, by utilizing the information found in this issue of *Physician Assistant Clinics*, we can have a tremendous impact on these numbers. While this issue of *Physician Assistant Clinics* focuses on endocrinology, the emphasis is on diabetes. As we all know, no matter what area we practice, there will always be a patient with diabetes, so this issue starts out with four great articles on the diagnosis, care, and treatment of the patient(s) with diabetes.

Ji Hyun Chun (CJ), the guest editor for this issue, has identified a number of great authors to provide us with the information we need to take care of these diabetic patients. This issue takes you from the diagnosis of diabetes with an article by O'Callaghan, to standards of care by Dugan, to treatment with an article on anti-hyperglycemic medications by Beer and special considerations in choosing therapy options (even a section on considering cost) for your diabetic patient by Murfin.

Not everything in endocrinology is diabetes. Let's not forget about the thyroid. Sadler provides an excellent review of the evaluation and workup of the patient with a thyroid nodule, and Bahroo looks at the utilization of the T3 test in the evaluation of patients with thyroid disease. But, it is the pituitary and adrenals that seem to give us all pause as we try to figure out the various tests we can order and treatment options. Pinkson provides an excellent review of pituitary disorders, including the various adenomas and their presentations, diabetes insipidus, and pituitary apoplexy. Scheckel provides the adrenal review. Her focus is on adrenal insufficiency, Cushing syndrome, and pheochromocytoma (after reading this you will be able to get right those one or two questions on pheochromocytoma that are on every PANCE and PANRE).

Physician Assist Clin 2 (2017) xi–xii
http://dx.doi.org/10.1016/j.cpha.2016.10.002
2405-7991/17/© 2016 Published by Elsevier Inc.

physicianassistant.theclinics.com

I hope you enjoy the fifth issue of *Physician Assistant Clinics*. Our next issue will provide you with a review of the latest in infectious disease.

Of note, this issue starts the second year of *Physician Assistant Clinics*. As consulting editor, I have had the pleasure to work with some wonderful guest editors and authors. Everyone I have reached out to has been happy to help, or at times happy to supply me names of others who can help. I hope the first year of the *Physician Assistant Clinics* has provided you with interesting and thorough articles that you can use in your practice or preparing for exams. If you have suggestions for enhancements or possible future topics, drop me a note at the e-mail below. Thank you, and I hope you continue to put us at the top of your reading list.

James Van Rhee, MS, PA-C
Yale University
Yale Physician Assistant Program
100 Church Street South, Suite A250
New Haven, CT 06519, USA

E-mail address:
james.vanrhee@yale.edu

REFERENCE

1. Centers for Disease Control and Prevention. National Diabetes Statistics Report: estimates of diabetes and its burden in the United States, 2014. Atlanta (GA): US Department of Health and Human Services; 2014.

Preface
Unraveling the Mystery of Endocrinology

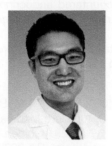

Ji Hyun Chun (CJ), MPAS, PA-C, BC-ADM
Editor

The field of endocrinology is viewed as one of the most convoluted fields of medicine. Compared with the other specialties, there are limited numbers of physician assistants practicing in endocrinology. With the shortage of supply of clinical endocrinologists, many referring providers and patients struggle to get in to see the endocrinologist in a timely manner. Therefore, it often falls back to the primary care providers to manage the patients' endocrinopathy, at least in the interim. Good understanding of the endocrine system will allow the clinicians to initiate the diagnostic process and sort out who truly needs further endocrine evaluation or who can be kept. It will also speed up the diagnostic process from endocrinologists' end when given appropriate initial workup that is already done because it often requires multiple laboratory values and stepwise evaluation.

The management of diabetes mellitus is absolutely the most common reason for the referral. Fortunately, there have been big advances in the understanding of the disease and its treatment options. However, it also has put a lot of pressure on clinicians to keep up with these changes, which often is not easy if one has to keep up with other fields of medicine as well. Therefore, almost 30% of the contents, 4 of 11 articles, are dedicated to diabetes management.

Along with diabetes, thyroid disorders are considered "bread and butter" in endocrinology. Most clinicians are comfortable with managing hypothyroidism, and most referrals for hypothyroidism are driven by the patients rather than the clinicians. T3 therapy remains controversial with big interest in some patients as well as clinicians. Thyrotoxicosis and nodular thyroid disorders often require endocrine referrals and are discussed here.

Obesity has become epidemic in the United States, and with its comorbidities, it will bankrupt the country if left alone. Many medical organizations are taking charge in battling this devastating and challenging disease, and physician assistants have to be on the frontline of this battle.

Physician Assist Clin 2 (2017) xiii–xiv
http://dx.doi.org/10.1016/j.cpha.2016.10.001
2405-7991/17/© 2016 Published by Elsevier Inc.

physicianassistant.theclinics.com

Pituitary and adrenal glands are possibly the reason some clinicians "fear" the field of endocrinology. Conversely, many clinicians chose endocrinology because of these hypothalamus-pituitary disorders. It will often require endocrine referral, but starting up the right diagnostic process while the patient is waiting for the first visit with the endocrinologist will shorten the time to the right diagnosis, which can make a world of difference to the patients.

Parathyroid and calcium disorders are commonly encountered endocrinopathies that can be enjoyable to come to the right diagnosis and treatment plan with good understanding of the physiology and pathophysiology.

It is my utmost pleasure to present you with our all-star authors well represented across the nation and diverse practice settings: private clinics, academic centers, and national health centers.

Ji Hyun Chun (CJ), MPAS, PA-C, BC-ADM
OptumCare Medical Group
30281 Golden Lantern
Laguna Niguel, CA 92677, USA

A.T. Still University
Mesa, AZ 85206, USA

E-mail address:
cjcmedicine@gmail.com

Diagnosing Diabetes Mellitus

Sondra O'Callaghan, PA-C, MPH, CHES

KEYWORDS

- Diabetes • Screening • Diagnosis • Classification • Autoimmune • Insulin resistance
- Gestational

KEY POINTS

- Screening and diagnosis—with the rising incidence and prevalence of diabetes, identification of individuals living with this problem is critical for possible prevention or early treatment.
- Correct classification—determination of the cause of diabetes or dysglycemia lends to a more thorough approach to the best care.
- Optimization of therapy—the cause of diabetes often dictates therapeutic choices, allowing for optimization of treatment, reduction of complications, and, ultimately, amelioration of disease burden.

INTRODUCTION

There is no debate regarding the massive disease burden imposed by diabetes mellitus. Evaluation of United States surveys of health data shows that from 2011 to 2012, the estimated prevalence of diabetes was 12% to 14% among US adults.[1] Statistics from the Centers for Disease Control and Prevention show the incidence in those 65 to 79 years of age nearly doubling from 1980 through 2014.[2] Further described is the impact on people aged 0 to 44 years of age who experienced a 217% increase in diagnosis of diabetes from 1990 to 2009.[3]

The United States is not the only country seeing dramatic changes in the rate of diagnosis of diabetes. The International Diabetes Federation estimates that by 2040, there will be more than 640 million people globally living with diabetes.[4] It follows that with more and more people living with diabetes for long periods of time, it is of great urgency to screen, diagnose, and classify correctly and, thereby, treat most appropriately for the best outcomes.

The author has no disclosures.
Division of Endocrinology, NF/SG Veterans Health System, 1601 Southwest Archer Road, 111B-1, Gainesville, FL 32608-1135, USA
E-mail address: acorporeal@comcast.net

Physician Assist Clin 2 (2017) 1–12
http://dx.doi.org/10.1016/j.cpha.2016.08.003
2405-7991/17/© 2016 Elsevier Inc. All rights reserved.

physicianassistant.theclinics.com

SCREENING

With increasing prevalence of diabetes and increased disease burden, identification of those individuals becomes paramount. The importance of screening, diagnosis, and subsequent correct classification is evidenced by the benefit conferred on a patient for (1) prevention, (2) risk stratification, (3) improved fetal outcomes, (4) prediction of disease state progression, and (5) impact on therapy.

Prevention

In terms of type 1 diabetes mellitus (T1D) prevention, studies are looking at primary and secondary prevention. Genetics, environment, and autoimmunity play a role in the development of T1D. Targeting gene expression, immune modulation, and environmental factors may ultimately lead to significant alteration in disease expression or progression. Primary prevention has focused on diet modification in those with genetic risk but without islet autoantibodies, whereas secondary prevention (or delay of onset) with pharmacotherapy has been studied in individuals with multiple islet autoantibodies but without hyperglycemia.[5]

Identifying people with abnormal glucose homeostasis is a strong strategy for disease prevention. The natural history of type 2 diabetes mellitus (T2D) is such that there exist abnormal glucoses years before disease diagnosis. It is well known that intervening in the earliest stages of glucose dysregulation can delay or even prevent progression to frank T2D. In the landmark Diabetes Prevention Program, the incidence of diabetes was reduced by 58% with lifestyle intervention and 31% with metformin therapy.[6] Despite having established guidelines for screening, diagnosis, and management of various states of hyperglycemia, only a small percentage of those eligible receive hemoglobin (A_{1c}) testing; application of screening guidelines could result in the detection of many cases of undiagnosed hyperglycemia.[7] Although many patients are recognized as having prediabetes (or even T2D), they often do not receive the appropriate care for prevention or treatment.[8,9]

Risk Stratification

In genetically susceptible individuals, islet autoantibodies are present months to years prior to development of symptoms and can aid in diagnosis and classification of T1D as well as identification of people at risk for disease development through detection in first-degree relatives.[5] In patients both genetically and immunologically predisposed to T1D, including latent autoimmune diabetes of adults (LADA), it has been theorized that identification of insulitis with imaging modalities and initiation of immunotherapy at an early, preclinical stage could modulate the autoimmune process.[10] Individuals with islet cell antibody positivity are prone to develop other autoimmune disorders, such as autoimmune thyroid disease, celiac disease, vitiligo, Addison disease, autoimmune hepatitis, myasthenia gravis, and pernicious anemia.[11] This association has also been observed to be true in individuals having LADA, where even low-titer glutamic acid decarboxylase antibody (GADA) positivity was associated with autoimmune thyroid disease.[12]

In individuals with other genetic forms of diabetes, for example, maturity-onset diabetes of the young (MODY), molecular genetic testing is recommended, because it predicts clinical course and defines risk in family members.[13,14] Furthermore, if an individual is found to have diabetes as a component of a syndrome, correct identification of the entity has implications for the individual and possibly family members.

For those at risk for T2D, earlier identification of prediabetes aids risk stratification. Even in this state, before formal diagnosis of diabetes, there is increased risk for atherosclerotic cardiovascular disease and microvascular complications (ie, retinopathy, neuropathy, and microalbuminuria)[15]; therefore, lifestyle and pharmacotherapies targeting glucose, lipid, and blood pressure levels are recommended.[16] There exists a strong genetic component to T2D, with 24 genetic foci associated with glycemic traits and 153 foci associated with risk of T2D; also identified are protective foci associated with T2D and glycemic traits.[17]

Improved Fetal Outcomes

It has been established that women with gestational diabetes mellitus (GDM) carry an increased risk for development of T2D later in life. It was not until 2008 that the Hyperglycemia and Adverse Pregnancy Outcome study[18] looked at perinatal outcomes in patients with hyperglycemia during pregnancy. It showed that maternal hyperglycemia (not severe enough to define as overt diabetes) is related to clinically important perinatal outcomes: birthweight above the 90th percentile, cord blood serum C-peptide level above the 90th percentile, primary cesarean delivery, neonatal hypoglycemia, premature delivery, shoulder dystocia/birth injury, intensive neonatal care, hyperbilirubinemia, and preeclampsia.

Prediction of Disease State Progression

Islet autoantibody positivity can portend β-cell decline.[19,20] It has been observed that there is a relationship between GADA titers and β-cell destruction, with higher GADA seen in individuals with β-cell failure.[12] It is suggested that autoantibodies drive the β-cell destruction with approximately 40% annual decline in β-cell function in those with autoimmune diabetes and 8% annual decline in those with nonautoimmune, insulin-resistant diabetes.[21] Correct classification of diabetes is important when there is little risk for disease progression, for example, individuals with type 2 MODY, which involves glucokinase mutation, have stable, mild fasting hyperglycemia over a lifetime without complications and do not warrant treatment.[22]

Impact on Therapy

Although this discussion is not regarding therapies for diabetes, it must be understood that some forms of diabetes are amenable to certain therapies, and elucidation of the correct cause can optimize care for the individual.

Populations to Be Screened

The American Diabetes Association (ADA) and the American Association of Clinical Endocrinologists recommend screening for asymptomatic adults who meet high-risk cardiovascular, metabolic, ethnic, and familial criteria, generally every 3 years starting at age 45 years. Screening starts sooner if the individual is overweight. Risk factors include the following: being overweight, being sedentary, having a first-degree relative with diabetes, GDM, delivery of baby more than 9 pounds, hypertension, high triglycerides, low high-density lipoprotein, cardiovascular disease, polycystic ovarian syndrome, insulin resistance, hemoglobin A_{1c} greater than 5.6% (prediabetes), high-risk race, or antipsychotic therapy.[23,24]

With the striking rise in T2D among children, it is important to identify this problem to achieve earlier diagnosis and implementation of therapy to reduce risk for complications.[25] The ADA recommends screening asymptomatic children less than or equal to 18 years of age for T2D if the child is overweight and has 2 risk factors, for example, family history, high-risk race, insulin resistance, or mother with GDM during child's gestation.[23] When evaluating hyperglycemia in children, however, etiologies of both T1D and T2D must be entertained.

It was not until 2011 that screening at 24 to 28 weeks of gestation was recommended for all pregnant women without known diabetes.[26] Currently, screening for GDM should be at the first prenatal visit and 24 to 28 weeks gestation by ADA guidelines.[23] It is further recommended that those individuals found to have GDM be screened 6 to 12 weeks postpartum using oral glucose tolerance test (OGTT) and subsequently screened lifelong every 3 years, because they are at increased risk of developing diabetes in the future.

Screening/Diagnostic Tools

In 2009, the International Expert Committee as well as the World Health Organization approved the use of hemoglobin A_{1c} as a diagnostic tool for diabetes with a cutpoint of 6.5%.[27,28] In 2010, the ADA added hemoglobin A_{1c} to recommended tests for diagnosis of diabetes.[29] Currently, fasting plasma glucose (FPG), 2-hour plasma glucose (PG) during OGTT, hemoglobin A_{1c}, and random PG with classic symptoms are tests used to diagnose diabetes. No one test is superior to the rest for diagnosis.[23]

DIAGNOSIS

The diagnosis of diabetes can be made by FPG greater than or equal to 126 mg/dL, 2-hour PG greater than or equal to 200 mg/dL during 75-g OGTT, hemoglobin A_{1c} greater than or equal to 6.5%, or random PG greater than or equal to 200 in the setting of hyperglycemic symptoms (**Fig. 1**). The first 3 tests require repeat confirmation in the absence of unequivocal hyperglycemia. The same test should be repeated to confirm the diagnosis. If 2 different tests are used and they are both above diagnostic threshold, diabetes is confirmed. If there is discordance between 2 tests, that is, one meets criteria whereas the other does not, the one that is above the diagnostic cutpoint should be repeated for diagnosis.[23]

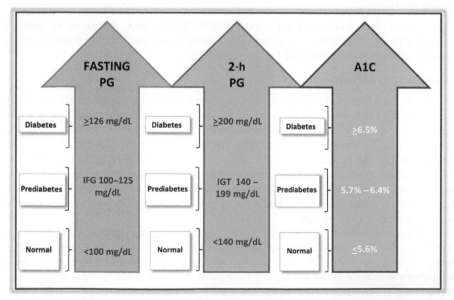

Fig. 1. Diagnostic criteria for diabetes and prediabetes. A1C, hemoglobin A_{1c}; IFG, impaired fasting glucose; IGT, impaired glucose tolerance.

CLASSIFICATION

Once an individual meets diagnostic criteria for diabetes, it is important to discern the cause. The impact of proper classification goes beyond satisfaction of academic knowledge. There exist implications for risk stratification, prediction of disease state progression, and therapy optimization. Elucidating etiology of dysglycemia can prove difficult. Although not entirely exhaustive, the etiologic classification of diabetes is outlined.

Type 1 Diabetes Mellitus

Immune-mediated diabetes mellitus

It is estimated that 5% to 10% of diabetes cases fall in the category of immune-mediated diabetes mellitus. Although it is most commonly diagnosed in children and the young, it can be diagnosed well into adulthood, even into the 8th and 9th decades of life. Individuals are prone to ketoacidosis, owing to insulin deficiency from β-cell destruction. It results from autoimmune destruction of β-cells marked by islet cell autoantibodies, strong HLA associations (which are inherited), and environmental factors.[23] The most common immune markers include islet cell autoantibodies, insulin autoantibodies, GADA, tyrosine phosphatases islet antigen antibodies (IA-2) and IA-2β, and zinc transporter 8.

Studies show that insulitis is present for months or even years in the preclinical stage of this disease.[10,30,31] Furthermore, it has been observed that blood glucose begins to increase at least 2 years before diagnosis and continues to increase gradually until at least 6 months before diagnosis, during which time there is a steeper rise in blood glucose.[32] The progression of this immune response happens sequentially and at a variable rate. For example, quicker progression to insulin dependency is seen in the presence of multiple autoantibodies and high titers of GADA.[19,33] In those diagnosed as adults (LADA), lower genetic load and subtle gene variations can be seen compared with the young with autoimmune diabetes,[34] lending to less aggressive β-cell loss.[33] Many adults, therefore, are misclassified as having T2D, because the rate of loss of β-cell function can be similar to that in T2D.[12] An individual may carry a diagnosis of T2D yet have immunogenetic characteristics of T1D.[35] It is now known that approximately 10% of adult diabetes is autoimmune,[20] and LADA is prevalent in China, more so than childhood-onset autoimmune diabetes.[36]

Idiopathic type 1 diabetes mellitus

Subsets of individuals with ketosis and no evidence of autoimmunity have been identified. The Osaka Study Group described a subtype of T1D with rapid onset of hyperglycemia and absence of diabetes-related antibodies.[37] For years, there have been observations of ketosis-prone African Americans, some of whom did not require insulin therapy indefinitely.[38] Studies of these typically multiethnic individuals have birthed a proposal for their classification: autoantibody positive, loss of β-cell functional reserve (A+β− group), autoantibody positive, preservation of β-cell functional reserve (A+ β+ group), autoantibody negative, loss of β-cell functional reserve (A−β− group), and autoantibody negative, preservation of β-cell functional reserve (A−β+ group).[39]

Type 2 Diabetes Mellitus

Approximately 90% to 95% of people with diabetes have the T2D form of diabetes, involving insulin resistance, which is the major etiologic defect. Insulin deficiency can be present secondary to defective β-cell function, although many do not require insulin therapy and most do not become ketotic. The early 1980s saw many studies beginning to elucidate the mechanisms of insulin resistance in patients with diabetes, including insulin receptor abnormalities,[40] hepatic and peripheral resistance to insulin action,[41] and insulin resistance involving multiple pathways in metabolism of glucose and lipids, with evidence that the dysregulation of glucose and lipid metabolism may be interrelated.[42]

There is a strong genetic component to the development of T2D (discussed previously). This is not well understood, however, and environmental factors also contribute. Overweight and physical inactivity are 2 environmental factors that play a key role in the development of insulin resistance and subsequent progression to diabetes. Not all individuals with T2D are overweight; it has been observed in the Asian Indian population, the major defect contributing diabetes is insulin resistance, often in the absence of obesity.[43]

Gestational Diabetes Mellitus

The gestational form of diabetes mellitus is first recognized during the second or third trimester of pregnancy; if it is discovered in the first trimester, it is considered T2D.[23] As described previously, treating maternal hyperglycemia improves fetal outcomes. Diagnosis can be made by differing strategies and diagnostic cutpoints (**Fig. 2**).[23,44,45]

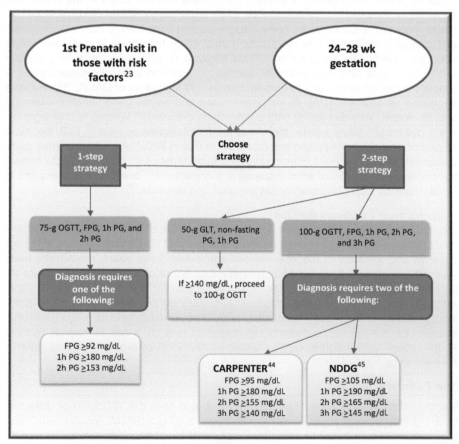

Fig. 2. Screening recommendations for GDM. 1h, 1-hour; 2h, 2-hour; 3h, 3-hour; GLT, glucose loading test; NDDG, National Diabetes Data Group. (*Data from* Refs.[23,44,45])

Diabetes Secondary to Genetics

The forms of secondary diabetes which are due to genetics are non-T1D and non-T2D and involve genetic mutations with effect on β-cell function or insulin action.

MODY has an autosomal dominant mode of transmission warranting genetic counseling and can exhibit abnormalities of β-cell function or insulin signaling.[13] Individuals with MODY are typically diagnosed with T1D or T2D, do not exhibit characteristics of either, are islet antibody negative, and have a strong family history of diabetes. Best practice guidelines for the molecular genetic diagnosis of MODY give the following clinical criteria for testing: mild fasting hyperglycemia, GDM with persistently elevated FPG after pregnancy, children/young adults with diabetes, and babies with diazoxide-responsive neonatal hyperinsulinemic hypoglycemia.[14] Knowledge of MODY type often determines treatment (**Fig. 3**).[14] Some MODY types respond well to sulfonylureas, others require only diet therapy, and others require insulin.[46]

Some forms of diabetes result from genetic defects in insulin action: leprechaunism, type A insulin resistance, Rabson-Mendenhall syndrome, and lipoatrophic diabetes.[47]

Maternally inherited diabetes and deafness (MIDD) is transmitted maternally and is associated with deafness and sometimes neurologic problems. Neonatal diabetes can result from one of several gene mutations, necessitating appropriate genetic diagnosis for optimal treatment.[17]

Many genetic syndromes (**Fig. 4**) are associated with diabetes by mechanisms affecting insulin secretion, insulin resistance, or glucose production.[48]

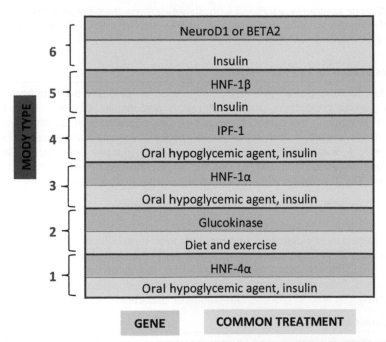

Fig. 3. MODY type and affected gene. BETA2, β-cell E-box transactivator 2; HNF-4α, hepatocyte nuclear factor; IPF, insulin promoter factor; NeuroD1, neurogenic differentiation factor 1. (*Data from* Fajans SS, Bell GI, Polonsky KS. Molecular mechanisms and clinical pathophysiology of maturity-onset diabetes of the young. N Engl J Med 2001;345(13):971–90.)

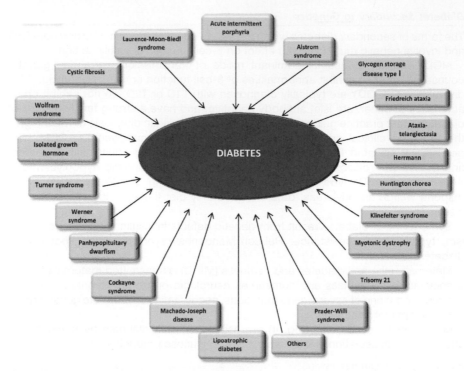

Fig. 4. Genetic syndromes associated with diabetes. (*Data from* Catanese VM. Secondary forms of diabetes. In: Skyler JS, editor. Atlas of diabetes. 3rd edition. Philadelphia: Current Medicine LLC; 2006. p. 241–51.)

Diabetes Secondary to Endocrinopathy

Secondary forms of diabetes can arise from endocrine diseases owing to hormone effect on glucose production, glucose utilization, and insulin secretion. The hormone involved determines the defect, for example, glucocorticoids in Cushing syndrome inhibit insulin secretion and impair insulin action, whereas excess catecholamine and thyroxine levels alter glucose production and glucose utilization.[48] Diabetes from these diseases often remits when the underlying disturbance of the disease is corrected. **Fig. 5** shows some endocrinopathies associated with diabetes.

Diabetes Secondary to Disorders of the Exocrine Pancreas

Diseases affecting the functional mass (involving approximately 75%) of the pancreas can cause secondary diabetes. Abnormal glucose metabolism is seen in hemochromatosis secondary to defective first-phase insulin secretion and hepatic insulin resistance.[48] In cystic fibrosis, insulin insufficiency is the primary etiologic defect of dysglycemia. Trauma, pancreatectomy, pancreatitis, neoplasia, and fibrocalcific pancreatopathy can lead to glucose intolerance or diabetes.[47]

Other Forms of Diabetes

Drugs or chemicals can change glucose homeostasis by altering insulin secretion or insulin action. Some of the types (**Fig. 6**) include but are not limited to adrenergics, anticonvulsants, antihelminthics, antihypertensives, blocking agents, cations, diuretics, hormones, pesticides, and psychopharmacologic agents.[48]

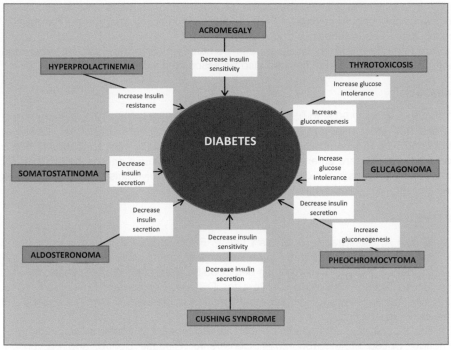

Fig. 5. Endocrinopathies associated with diabetes. (*Data from* Catanese VM. Secondary forms of diabetes. In: Skyler JS, editor. Atlas of diabetes. 3rd edition. Philadelphia: Current Medicine LLC; 2006.)

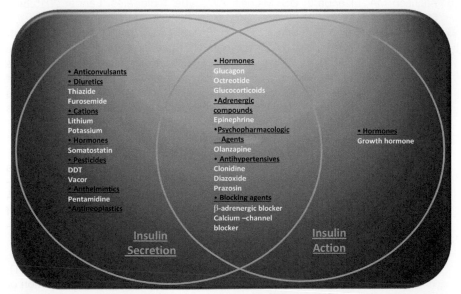

Fig. 6. Pharmacologic effects of drugs on glucose disposition. (*Data from* Catanese VM. Secondary forms of diabetes. In: Skyler JS, editor. Atlas of diabetes. 3rd edition. Philadelphia: Current Medicine LLC; 2006.)

Infections have been implicated in the development of diabetes associated with effect on β-cell function. Some of these include cytomegalovirus, congenital rubella, coxsackievirus B, adenovirus, and mumps.[47]

Rare immune-mediated diseases, stiff person syndrome (high GADA titers), and anti-insulin receptor antibodies can also be associated with diabetes.[47]

SUMMARY

With approximately 90% to 95% of people with diabetes having T2D, it is often presumed that most new cases are such. There are various mechanisms, however, that contribute to the impairment of glucose homeostasis leading to diabetes. Some forms of diabetes are amenable to certain therapies. Cause can be determined for appropriate diagnosis and classification, and, in turn, individuals living with diabetes can benefit from optimal care tailored to their needs.

REFERENCES

1. Menke A, Casagrande S, Geiss L, et al. Prevalence of and trends in diabetes among adults in the United States, 1988-2012. JAMA 2015;314(10):1021–9.
2. Incidence of diagnosed diabetes per 1,000 population aged 18-79 years, by age, United States, 1980-2014. Centers for Disease Control and Prevention; 2015. Available at: www.cdc.gov/diabetes/statistics/incidence/fig3.htm. Accessed April 21, 2016.
3. Rates of diagnosed diabetes per 100 civilian, non-institutionalized population, by age, United States, 1980-2014. Centers for Disease Control and Prevention; 2015. Available at: www.cdc.gov/diabetes/statistics/prev/national/figpersons. htm. Accessed March 21, 2016.
4. IDF diabetes atlas-seventh edition 2015. International Diabetes Federation website. Available at: www.diabetesatlas.org. Accessed March 16, 2016.
5. Atkinson MA, Eisenbarth GS, Michels AW. Type 1 diabetes. Lancet 2015;383: 69–82.
6. Diabetes Prevention Program Research Group. Reduction in the incidence of Type 2 diabetes with lifestyle or metformin. N Engl J Med 2002;346:393–403.
7. Sohler N, Matti-Orozco B, Young E, et al. Opportunistic screening for diabetes and prediabetes using hemoglobin a1c in an urban primary care setting. Endocr Pract 2016;22(2):143–50.
8. Mainous AG III, Tanner RJ, Baker R. Prediabetes diagnosis and treatment in primary care. J Am Board Fam Med 2016;29(2):283–5.
9. Clark NG. Standards of care in diabetes. In: Leahy JL, Clark NG, Cefalu WT, editors. Medical management of diabetes Mellitus. New York: Marcel Dekker; 2000. p. 41–9.
10. Signore A, Capriotti G, Chianelli M, et al. Detection of insulitis by pancreatic scintigraphy with 99mTc-labeled IL-2 and MRI in patients with LADA (action LADA 10). Diabetes Care 2015;38(4):652–8.
11. Baker JR. Autoimmune endocrine disease. JAMA 1985;278(22):1931–7.
12. Liu L, Xiang Y, Huang G, et al. Latent autoimmune diabetes in adults with Low-titer GAD antibodies: similar disease progression with Type 2 diabetes. A nationwide, multicenter prospective study (LADA China 3). Diabetes Care 2015;38(1): 16–21.
13. Fajans SS, Bell GI, Polonsky KS. Molecular mechanisms and clinical pathophysiology of maturity-onset diabetes of the young. N Engl J Med 2001;345(13): 971–90.

14. Ellard S, Bellanne-Chantelot C, Hattersley AT. Best practice guidelines for the molecular genetic diagnosis of maturity-onset diabetes of the young. Diabetologia 2008;51(4):546–53.
15. Garber AJ, Handelsman Y, Einhorn D, et al. Diagnosis and management of prediabetes in the continuum of hyperglycemia-when do the risks of diabetes begin? A consensus statement from the American College of Endocrinology and the American Association of Clinical Endocrinologists. Endocr Pract 2008;14(7): 933–46.
16. Garber AJ, Abrahamson MJ, Barzilay JI, et al. Consensus statement by the American Association of Endocrinologists and American College of Endocrinology on the comprehensive type 2 diabetes management algorithm-2016 executive summary. Endocr Pract 2016;22(1):84–102.
17. Prasad RB, Groop L. Genetics of type 2 diabetes-pitfalls and possibilities. Genesis 2015;6(1):87–123.
18. The HAPO Study Cooperative Research Group, Metzger BE, Lowe LP, Dyer AR, et al. Hyperglycemia and adverse pregnancy outcomes. N Engl J Med 2008; 358(19):1991–2002.
19. Merger SR, Leslie RD, Boehm BO. The broad clinical phenotype of type 1 diabetes at presentation. Diabet Med 2012;30(2):170–8.
20. Hawa MI, Kolb H, Schloot N, et al. Adult-onset autoimmune diabetes in europe is prevalent with a broad clinical phenotype. Diabetes Care 2013;36(4):908–13.
21. Dabelea D, Mayer-Davis EJ, Andrews JS, et al. Clinical evolution of beta cell function in youth with diabetes: the SEARCH for Diabetes in Youth Study. Diabetologia 2012;55(12):3359–68.
22. Ellard S, Beards F, Allen LIS, et al. A high prevalence of glucokinase mutations in gestational diabetic subjects selected by clinical criteria. Diabetologia 2000; 43(2):250–3.
23. American Diabetes Association. Standards of medical care in Diabetes-2016. Diabetes Care 2016;39(Supp 1):S13–22.
24. Handelsman Y, Bloomgarden ZT, Grunberger G, et al. American Association of Clinical Endocrinologists and American College of Endocrinology – clinical practice guidelines for developing a diabetes mellitus comprehensive care plan. Endocr Pract 2015;21(suppl 1):1–87.
25. Rodbard HW. Diabetes screening, diagnosis, and therapy in pediatric patients with Type 2 Diabetes. Medscape J Med 2008;10(8):184.
26. American Diabetes Association. Standards of medical care in Diabetes-2011. Diabetes Care 2011;34(Supp 1):S11–61.
27. International Expert Committee. International Expert Committee report on the role of the A1c assay in the diagnosis of diabetes. Diabetes Care 2009;32:1327–34.
28. World Health Organization. Use of glycated haemoglobin (HbA1c) in the diagnosis of diabetes Mellitus: abbreviated report of a WHO consultation. Geneva (Switzerland): World Health Org; 2009.
29. American Diabetes Association. Standards of medical care in diabetes-2010. Diabetes Care 2010;33(Supp 1):S62–9.
30. Botazzo GF, Dean BM, McNally JM, et al. In situ characterization of autoimmune phenomena and expression of hla molecules in the pancreas in diabetic insulitis. N Engl J Med 1985;313(6):353–60.
31. Eisenbarth GS. Type 1 Diabetes mellitus: a chronic autoimmune disease. N Engl J Med 1986;314(21):1360–8.

32. Sosenko JM, Palmer JP, Greenbaum CJ, et al. Patterns of metabolic progression to type 1 diabetes in the diabetes prevention trial-Type 1. Diabetes Care 2006; 29(3):643–9.
33. Laugesen E, Osteergaard JA, Leslie RDG. Latent autoimmune diabetes of the adult: current knowledge and uncertainty. Diabet Med 2015;32(7):843–52.
34. Howson JMM, Rosinger S, Smyth DJ, et al. Genetic analysis of adult-onset auto-immune diabetes. Diabetes 2011;60(10):2645–53.
35. Leslie RD, Palmer J, Schloot N. Diabetes at the crossroads: relevance of disease classification to pathophysiology and treatment. Diabetologia 2015;59(1):13–20.
36. Zhou Z, Xiang Y, Ji L, et al. Frequency, immunogenetics, and clinical character-istics of latent autoimmune diabetes in china (LADA China Study). Diabetes 2013;62(2):543–50.
37. Imagawa A, Hanafusa T, Miyagawa J, et al. A novel subtype of type 1 diabetes mellitus Characterized by a rapid onset and an absence of diabetes-related an-tibodies. N Engl J Med 2000;342(5):301–7.
38. Umpierrez GE, Casals MM, Gebhart SP. Diabetic ketoacidosis in obese African-Americans. Diabetes 1995;44(7):790–5.
39. Maldonado M, Hampe CS, Gaur LK, et al. Ketosis-prone diabetes: dissection of a heterogeneous syndrome using an immunogenetic and β-Cell functional classifi-cation, prospective analysis, and clinical outcomes. J Clin Endocrinol Metab 2003;88(11):5090–8.
40. Kolterman OG, Gray RS, Griffin J, et al. Receptor and postreceptor defects contribute to the insulin resistance in noninsulin-dependent diabetes mellitus. J Clin Invest 1981;68(4):957–69.
41. DeFronzo RA, Simonson D, Ferrannini E. Hepatic and peripheral insulin resis-tance: a common feature of type 2 (non-insulin-dependent) and type 1 (insulin-dependent) diabetes mellitus. Diabetologia 1982;23(4):313–9.
42. Groop LC, Bonadonna RC, DelPrato S, et al. Glucose and free fatty acid meta-bolism in non-insulin-dependent diabetes mellitus. Evidence for multiple sites of insulin resistance. J Clin Invest 1989;84(1):205–13.
43. Abate N, Chandalia M. Ethnicity and type 2 diabetes: focus on Asian Indians. J Diabetes Complications 2001;15(6):320–7.
44. Carpenter MW, Coustan DR. Criteria for screening tests for gestational diabetes. Am J Obstet Gynecol 1982;144(7):768–73.
45. National Diabetes Data Group. Classification and diagnosis of diabetes mellitus and other categories of glucose intolerance. Diabetes 1979;28(12):1039–57.
46. Fajans SS, Bell GI. MODY History, genetics, pathophysiology, and clinical deci-sion making. Diabetes Care 2011;34(8):1878–84.
47. American Diabetes Association. Standards of medical care in Diabetes-2014. Diabetes Care 2014;37(Supp 1):S14–80.
48. Catanese VM. Secondary forms of diabetes. In: Skyler JS, editor. Atlas of dia-betes. 3rd edition. Philadelphia: Current Medicine LLC; 2006. p. 241–51.

Standards of Care and Treatment in Diabetes

Joy A. Dugan, MPH, MSPAS, PA-C

KEYWORDS

- Diabetes mellitus • Guidelines • ADA • AACE

KEY POINTS

- Glucose control is only one factor in diabetes care. Blood pressure regulation, lipid control, weight management, and vaccinations all contribute to diabetes management.
- Individualize diabetes targets for patients based on age, activity, and comorbidities. Intensive management of diabetes raises the risk of hypoglycemia. Patients should only meet hemoglobin A1c targets if there is no considerable hypoglycemia.
- Refer for behavioral support when comorbid depression or diabetes distress exists. The Problem Area in Diabetes or the Diabetes Distress Scale can be used to facilitate this discussion.
- Smoking cessation, regular exercise, nutrition, and weight control are essential components to the treatment of diabetes.

INTRODUCTION

This article discusses the American Association of Clinical Endocrinologist/American College of Endocrinologists (AACE/ACE)[1] and American Diabetes Association (ADA)[2] 2016 guidelines for managing diabetes mellitus types 1 (T1DM) and 2 (T2DM). Although these guidelines exist, recognize that patients must also have individualized targets based on age, activity level, and comorbidity status. Furthermore, glucose control does not equate to diabetes control, because there are multiple other process and outcome measures, including blood pressure (BP), lipid, and weight control that contribute to successful diabetes management.

For all patients with diabetes, lifestyle optimization is key.[1,2] The AACE/ACE and ADA guidelines recommend frequently evaluating patients until stable using glycosylated hemoglobin A1c and self-monitored fasting and postprandial blood glucose levels. Weight changes, hypoglycemic events, exercise, cholesterol, BP, diabetes complications, comorbidities, drug reactions, and psychosocial factors should also be considered during a follow-up visit. Less frequent office visits should only occur once target measures are achieved.[1,2]

The author has nothing to disclose.
Joint MSPAS/MPH Program, Touro University California, 1310 Johnson Lane, Mare Island, CA 94592, USA
E-mail address: joy.dugan@tu.edu

Physician Assist Clin 2 (2017) 13–23
http://dx.doi.org/10.1016/j.cpha.2016.08.004
2405-7991/17/

STANDARDS OF CARE
Glycemic Control Targets

Glycemic targets are based on landmark trials including the Diabetes Control and Complications Trial (DCCT)[3] and The Epidemiology of Diabetes Interventions and Complications[3] for type 1 diabetes (T1DM) and the United Kingdom Prospective Diabetes Study (UKPDS)[4] for type 2 diabetes. These trials demonstrated that a reduction in blood glucose reduces the risk of microvascular complications.[3,4] In DCCT, individuals in the intensive therapy arm had a median A1c of 7% resulting in 35% to 76% reduction in early microvascular disease compared with the control group with a median A1c of 9%.[3] Similarly, UKPDS determined an A1c <7% led to fewer microvascular complications.[4] The AACE/ACE and ADA guidelines discussed later are based on these landmark trials.

Glycemic control for self-monitoring includes targets for both fasting and postprandial glucose states.[1,2] Guidelines by both AACE/ACE and ADA suggest first considering the patient's risk factors and comorbidities when establishing a treatment goal.[1,2] **Table 1** demonstrates the glycemic recommendations for patients with T1DM and type 2 diabetes (T2DM) where the AACE/ACE guidelines recommend more intensive goals than the ADA. The AACE/ACE support an A1c goal of 6.5% or less for most nonpregnant patients, whereas the ADA recommends an A1c goal of less than 7.0%. The lower AACE/ACE A1c goal is based on the landmark clinical trials, including DCCT and UKPDS, where microvascular complications can be reduced or prevented with even lower glycemic targets.[3,4]

In 2009, 3 trials, including Action in Diabetes and Vascular Disease Preterax and Diamicron MR Controlled Evaluation (ADVANCE) trial,[5] Action to Control Cardiovascular Risk in Diabetes (ACCORD),[6] and Veterans Affairs Diabetes Trials (VADT),[7] studied the effects of glycemic control on cardiovascular events. Both ADVANCE and VADT showed neutral effect on macrovascular complications with tight glycemic control in older

Table 1
Summary of American Association of Clinical Endocrinologist/American College of Endocrinologists and American Diabetes Association guidelines for glucose control

	AACE/ACE	ADA
Nonpregnant adult A1c goal	<6.5%	A1c goal of <7% with more stringent A1c (eg, <6.5%) if possible[a]
A1c goal with history of severe hypoglycemia, limited life expectancy, or extensive complications	<7%–8%	<8%
Preprandial capillary plasma glucose	<110	80–130 mg/dL
Postprandial capillary plasma glucose	<140	<180 mg/dL
Preexisting T1DM or T2DM who become pregnant	• Fasting 60–99 • Postprandial 100–129 • A1c <6.0%[a]	• Fasting 60–99 • Postprandial 100–129 • A1c <6.0%[a]

[a] If can be achieved without significant hypoglycemia.
Data from Garber AJ, Barzilay JI, Blonde L, et al. Consensus statement by the American Association of Clinical Endocrinologists and American College of Endocrinology on the comprehensive type 2 diabetes management algorithm—2016 executive summary. Endocr Pract 2016;22(1):84–113. Available at: https://www.aace.com/ sites/all/files/diabetes-algorithm-executive-summary.pdf.

patients with established cardiovascular disease.[5,7] In the ACCORD trial,[6] an increased mortality with tight glycemic control occurred among the frailest patients. Based on these trials, the ADA and AACE recommend individualizing targets for patients.

If a lower A1c cannot be achieved without adverse outcomes, then a goal of greater than 6.5% but up to 8% can be individualized per AACE/ACE. Because hypoglycemia risk increases with intensive glycemic control,[3,4,6] adjustments to the A1c goal may occur.[1] For patients with a history of severe hypoglycemia, short life expectancy, macrovascular complications, and other major comorbid conditions, a higher A1c may be more appropriate given the absence of hyperglycemia-associated symptoms (eg, polyuria, polydipsia, polyphagia).[1,2,6] The A1c recommendations for less intensive management are

- AACE/ACE: 7% to 8%
- ADA: less than 8%.

When possible, maximizing treatment is important, because both the DCCT and the UKPDS trials demonstrated intensive glucose control decreased the risk and progression of multiple microvascular complications associated with diabetes, such as nephropathy, neuropathy, and retinopathy.[3,4] Ultimately, managing the risk of hypoglycemia with the long-term effects of hyperglycemia is essential for patient safety, overall medical cost, and mortality; risk should be accounted for when determining glucose targets and A1c goals.[1,2]

WEIGHT CONTROL AND OBESITY MANAGEMENT

The ADA recommends at every office encounter that the patient's body mass index (BMI) be calculated and documented.[2] AACE/ACE recommends an overweight patient's weight be reassessed ideally every 3 months until improvements in weight loss occur.[1] The ADA and AACE/ACE recommend overweight (BMI of 25–29.9 kg/m^2) or obese (BMI $\geq$30 kg/m^2) patients reduce their body weight by 5% to 10% through decreased caloric intake and increased physical activity. Patients should strive for 500 to 750 calories per day energy deficit to achieve weight loss with a reduction in total calories as well as total saturated fat and sodium.[2] Patients should maintain a plant-based diet and be trained in meal planning, grocery shopping, and dining out, with a focus on limiting high-glycemic index foods, and if using insulin, match carbohydrate intake with insulin doses.[1] Decreases in A1c of 0.3% to 1% in patients with T1DM[8,9] and 0.5% to 2% in T2DM[2,10] can occur when medical nutrition therapy is delivered by a registered dietician. Sustained weight loss of greater than 7% is optimal.[2] Attending shared medical visits or diabetes self-management classes is especially helpful at delivering this lifestyle information.

In patients with comorbidities and a BMI greater than 27 kg/m,[2] weight-loss medications can be prescribed. **Box 1** lists the US Food and Drug Administration (FDA) -approved weight loss medications as of 2015.[1] The long-term FDA-approved medications for weight loss show a statically significant weight loss of up to 9.7% after 1 year of treatment.[1] For adult patients with a BMI $\geq$35 kg/m^2 and comorbidities, bariatric surgery should be considered, especially if goals have not been reached with other treatment options.[1,2] Bariatric surgery may also be helpful at addressing other comorbidities, including hypertension and obstructive sleep apnea. **Table 2** depicts a summary of treatment for overweight and obese patients with T2DM.[1,2]

HYPERTENSION MANAGEMENT AND RECOMMENDATIONS

The guidelines for hypertension in diabetes vary between Joint National Committee-8 (JNC-8), ADA, and AACE/ACE, as depicted in **Table 3**. The 2014 JNC-8 guidelines

---

Box 1
List of 2015 US Food and Drug Administration approved weight loss medications

Short term (few weeks)

Diethylproprion

Phendimetrazine

Long term

Liraglutide 3 mg

Lorcaserin

Naltrexone/buproprion

Orlistat

Phentermine/topirmate extended release

---

recommended less intensive BP management than previous JNC guidelines.[11] This recommendation is based on large-scale dating showing systolic BP less than 130 mm Hg does not reduce atherosclerotic cardiovascular disease (ASCVD) outcomes, and diastolic BP less than 70 mm Hg is associated with higher mortality.[3] In addition, results of the ACCORD Blood Pressure trial demonstrated reduction in cerebrovascular accidents and microalbuminuria with more intensive goals but no significant differences in cardiovascular or all-cause mortality.[6]

The angiotensin-converting enzyme inhibitor or angiotensin receptor blocker (ARB) is considered the medication of choice by the AACE/ACE and ADA for hypertension control in diabetes patients.[1,2] AACE/ACE and JNC-8 supports selection of any BP medication should be based on underlying factors such as history of myocardial infarction, congestive heart failure, and race/ethnicity.[1,11] The JNC-8 recommends choosing an angiotensin-converting enzyme inhibitor, ARB, calcium-channel blocker (CCB), or thiazide diuretic as first line for treating hypertension in both patients with and without diabetes.[11] In the African American hypertensive population, first-line classes are CCB or thiazide-type diuretics.[11]

Physician assistants should consider polypharmacy and side effects when prescribing any medications, including antihypertensive medications. Intensive therapy will require more antihypertensive medications, which previously were shown to incur

---

Table 2
Summary of treatment for overweight and obesity in type 2 diabetes from American Diabetes Association (2016)

Treatment	BMI Category (kg/m²)				
	23 (Asian Americans) 25.0–26.9	27.0–29.9	30.0–34.9	35.0–39.9	≥40
Lifestyle changes (diet, physical activity/exercise, and behavioral therapy)	X	X	X	X	X
Pharmacotherapy	—	X	X	X	X
Bariatric surgery	—	—	—	X	X

Adapted from American Diabetes Association. Obesity management for the treatment of type 2 diabetes. Diabetes Care 2016;39(Suppl 1):S47–51.

Table 3
Blood pressure guidelines by Joint National Committee-8, American Diabetes Association, and American Association of Clinical Endocrinologist/American College of Endocrinologists

JNC-8	
60 y or older	<150/90 mm Hg
59–30 y	Diastolic goal <90 mm Hg; insufficient evidence to recommend a systolic BP goal; panel recommends following expert opinion of 140/90 mm Hg
Hypertensive adult with diabetes and/or chronic kidney disease	140/90 mm Hg based on expert opinion
ADA	
General recommendation	<140/90 mm Hg
Younger, albuminuria, more risk factors	<130/80 mm Hg
AACE/ACE	
General recommendation	<130/80 mm Hg[a]
Individuals who can safely reach this target without side effects from medications	<120/80 mm Hg

[a] Obtain this goal when possible. This target goal can be less stringent if the patient has multiple other comorbidities (eg, frailty, adverse medication effects).
   Data from Refs.[1,2,11]

more adverse events and economic cost.[1] In addition to pharmacologic control, the AACE/ACE and ADA recommend patients restrict sodium following The Dietary Approaches to Stop Hypertension (DASH) diet. Following the low-sodium and high-potassium diet of the DASH diet can be safely recommended for all patients with diabetes mellitus in the absence of renal insufficiency.[2] Exercise should be recommended as a measure to help with both diabetes mellitus and BP control.[1] Early intervention is a hallmark in diabetes management; thus, the ADA recommends health care professionals discuss healthy lifestyle choices such as the DASH diet in individuals with a BP greater than 120/80 mm Hg.

ATHEROSCLEROTIC CARDIOVASCULAR DISEASE PREVENTION AND CHOLESTEROL MANAGEMENT
Cholesterol Management

Patients with diabetes have an increased risk of ASCVD, which includes acute coronary syndrome, history of myocardial infarction, angina, arterial revascularization, cerebral vascular disease, or transient ischemic attack.[1,2,12] The American College of Cardiology/American Heart Association (ACC/AHA) 2013 Guidelines for managing lipids recommend individuals with diabetes from 40 to 75 years old begin a moderate-to high-intensity statin to lower their ASCVD risk.[12] For individuals under age 40, consider additional risk factors before initiating statin therapy, including patient preference, potential for polypharmacy and drug-to-drug interactions, and management of other risk factors for ASCVD. Among the under-40 population, intensive lifestyle counseling should be considered to mitigate risk for ASCVD.

Individuals over 75 years of age with diabetes, the decision to start a statin should be individualized based on other risk factors.[2,12] This individualization should include their 10-year life expectancy, increased polypharmacy, and potential for interactions between drugs. **Box 2** depicts the AHA/ACC guideline for initiating statin therapy in patients with diabetes.

Box 2
Algorithm for managing cholesterol according to 2013 American Heart Association/American College of Cardiology Lifestyle Management Guidelines for patients with diabetes

LDL-C 70 to 189 mg/dL age 40 to 75 years

- Start moderate intensity statin

- Start high intensity statin if 10-year ASCVD risk ≥7.5%

LDL-C less than 70 mg/dL age less than 40 or greater than 75 years

- Consider statin therapy in select individuals

- Consider other factors including risk-reduction benefit, possible drug-to-drug interactions, and potential for adverse effects, and patient's choice

Data from Robinson JG, Stone NJ. The 2013 ACC/AHA guideline on the treatment of blood cholesterol to reduce atherosclerotic cardiovascular disease risk: a new paradigm supported by more evidence. Eur Heart J 2015;36(31):2110–8.

Instead of treating to target numbers, the updated ACC/AHA recommend reducing the low-density lipoprotein cholesterol (LDL-C) by an individualized percentage based on ASCVD risk score.[12] This risk score can be calculated using the ASCVD risk calculator (http://my.americanheart.org). **Table 4** shows the available statin therapies divided into intensity groups with dosage. Individuals with diabetes and greater than 7.5% estimated 10-year ASCVD risk should take a high-intensity statin. The AACE/ACE 2016 guidelines continue to set targets for cholesterol numbers (**Table 5**).[1]

The ACC/AHA 2013 guidelines do not include medication classes such as niacin, fenofibrates, and ezetimibe. For select patients at high risk for cardiovascular complications, the IMPROVE IT trial showed additional cardiovascular benefit when adding ezetimibe (Zetia) to a moderate-intensity statin. In addition, ezetimibe can be considered in selected patients who cannot tolerate high-intensity statin or needs additional LDL reduction.[13]

Aspirin Therapy

The AACE/ACE, ADA, and US Preventive Services Task Force recommend aspirin therapy for prevention of cardiovascular disease starting at age 50 to 59.[2,14] Aspirin

Table 4
Statin dosage and intensity

Intensity with Definition	Dosage
Low Daily dose lowers LDL-C by average <30%	Fluvastatin 20–40 mg Lovastatin 20 mg Pitavastatin 1 mg Pravastatin 10–20 mg Simvastatin 10 mg

Moderate
   Daily dose lowers LDL-C by approximately
      ≥30%-50%
	Atorvastatin 10–20 mg
	Fluvastatin 40 mg bid or Fluvastatin XL 80 mg qd
	Lovastatin 40 mg
	Pitavastatin 2–4 mg
	Pravastatin 40–80 mg
	Rosuvastatin 5–10 mg
	Simvastatin 20–40 mg

High Daily dose lowers the LDL-C on average ≥50%	Atorvastatin 40–80 mg Rosuvastatin 20–40 mg

Table 5
American Association of Clinical Endocrinologist/American College of Endocrinologists guidelines for lipids in patients with type 2 diabetes mellitus

	AACE/ACE Guidelines	
Cholesterol Marker	High-Risk Patients (T2DM but No Other Major Risk and/or Age <40 y)	Very High-Risk Patients (T2DM Plus >1 Major ASVD Risk or Established ASCVD)
LDL-C (mg/dL)	<100	<70
Non-high-density lipoprotein cholesterol (mg/dL)	<130	<100
Triglycerides (mg/dL)	<150	<150
Apo B (mg/dL)	<90	<80
LDL-P (nmol/L)	<1200	<1000
High-density lipoprotein	—	—

Adapted from Garber AJ, Barzilay JI, Blonde L, et al. Consensus statement by the American Association of Clinical Endocrinologists and American College of Endocrinology on the comprehensive type 2 diabetes management algorithm—2016 executive summary. Endocr Pract 2016;22:84–113.

therapy (75–162 mg/d) should be considered in both women and men with T1DM or T2DM.[2] Patients younger than 50 years with multiple risk factors including a history of ASCVD should consider aspirin therapy as secondary prevention.[15]

IMMUNIZATION

AACE/ACE and ADA support the Centers for Disease Control and Prevention's immunization recommendation for adults as depicted in the recommended adult immunization schedule for adults aged 19 years or older, by vaccine and age group. Available at: https://www.cdc.gov/vaccines/schedules/downloads/adult/adult-schedule.pdf.[1,2,16] Individuals with diabetes should receive routine immunizations for children and adults, including yearly influenza vaccine. In addition, hepatitis B vaccine should be administered to all unvaccinated adults aged 19 to 59 years. For individuals over the age of 60, consider administering the hepatitis B vaccine, especially if there are other risk factors for acquiring hepatitis B.

Exercise and Physical Activity

According to the American College of Sports Medicine/ADA guidelines of 2010, which are endorsed by AACE/ACE,[1] individuals with diabetes should achieve a minimum of

- Moderate intensity exercise for 150 minutes per week at 50% to 70% of the maximum heart rate (eg, walking briskly for 3 miles per hour or faster, water aerobics, bicycling about 10 miles per hour, doubles tennis, and gardening)
- Strength training at least twice weekly working most all the major muscle groups (eg, any modifications to squats, pushups, crunches, calf raises).
- Regular flexibility training (eg, yoga, tai chi, Pilates).[17]

Individuals should begin any new activity slowly and increase intensity and duration, as they are able to do so. The intensity of the exercise can be increased as the individual's fitness capacity increases.

Although patients with diabetes should be assessed if they are going to engage in more vigorous exercise than walking, there is no need for all patients with diabetes to undergo cardiac testing. A graded stress test should only be performed in symptomatic patients with cardiovascular disease risk factors.[17–20] Although higher levels of exercise intensity are associated with the greatest improvements of A1c,[1] recognize that some patients will need modifications to their exercise regimens if significant comorbidities exist. These comorbidities include the following:

- Unstable angina
- End-stage renal failure on dialysis
- Insulin pump use
- Peripheral neuropathy
- Charcot foot
- Peripheral arterial disease
- Proliferative retinopathy
- Macular degeneration[17,18]

Thus, physician assistants should regularly work with the diabetes health care team to include ophthalmologist and podiatrist to establish individualized and safe exercise and physical activity programming.

BEHAVIORAL SUPPORT

Diabetes is associated with higher rates of depression compared with the general population.[21] Assessing patients routinely for depression is important because approximately 20% or more of individuals with diabetes also suffer from depression.[1] An initial evaluation could be a part of the medical assistant's vital sign assessment. The medical assistant could ask the questions from the Patient Health Questionnaire-2, which includes the questions: (1) Do you ever feel hopeless, down, or depressed, and (2) Do you have little pleasure or interest in doing things you previously enjoyed?

Diabetes-related distress, which is the negative psychological reactions related to diabetes management, should be evaluated. Diabetes distress is not depression but instead the psychological response to managing a chronic disease. The Problem Area in Diabetes or the Diabetes Distress Scale can be used to facilitate this discussion and identify individuals with high levels of diabetes-related distress.[22,23] Identifying individuals with higher distress levels is important for long-term management of diabetes. Those with higher levels of diabetes distress have lower adherence to self-management behaviors, including physical activity and glucose monitoring.[24]

Managing a chronic disease such as diabetes can require a significant amount of psychosocial support for some patients. Encourage patients to join community groups, attend shared office or group visits, or support groups.[1,2] The ADA recommends referring patients who experience difficulty managing the stress associated with diabetes, other comorbid mental health disorders, possibility of self-harm or harm to others.[1]

SMOKING CESSATION

Both the ADA and the AACE/ACE recommend patients receive smoking cessation counseling and avoid all tobacco products.[1,2] Structured programs should be recommended for patients unable to stop smoking on their own.[2] Electronic cigarettes should not be recommended as a means of smoking cessation.[2] Instead, recommend FDA-approved medications to aid in smoking cessation as depicted in **Box 3**.[25]

Box 3
US Food and Drug Administration–approved smoking cessation medications

Over-the-counter smoking cessation medications

Nicotine replacement
    Nicotine patches
    Nicotine gum
    Nicotine lozenges

Prescription smoking cessation medications

Nicotine replacement
    Nicotine inhaler spray
    Nicotine nasal spray

Nicotine withdrawal reduction
    Buproprion (Zyban)
    Varenicline (Chantix)

SUMMARY

Although 2 guidelines exist for diabetes management, the overall intent of both ADA and AACE/ACE guidelines is to reduce the complications from diabetes mellitus. Based on landmark trials, the current guidelines seek to minimize microvascular complications and improve morbidity for individuals with diabetes. Intensive lifestyle management through regular exercise, weight control, and nutrition is the hallmark of diabetes management. Although lacking consensus with regards to specific goals, hypertension and hyperlipidemia should be treated to avoid potential sequela from ASCVD. The physician assistant should consider adjunctive therapies, such as smoking cessation counseling, behavioral counseling, and medical nutrition therapy, to optimize diabetes therapies when appropriate.

REFERENCES

1. Garber AJ, Barzilay JI, Blonde L, et al. Consensus statement by the American Association of Clinical Endocrinologists and American College of Endocrinology on the comprehensive type 2 diabetes management algorithm—2016 executive summary. Endocr Pract 2016;22(1):84–113. Available at: https://www.aace.com/sites/all/files/diabetes-algorithm-executive-summary.pdf.

2. American Diabetes Association. Standards of medical care in diabetes—2016. Diabetes Care 2016;39(S1).

3. Nathan DM. The diabetes control and complications trial/epidemiology of diabetes interventions and complications study at 30 years: overview. Diabetes Care 2014;27(1):9–16.

4. King P, Peacock I, Donnelly R. The UK prospective diabetes study (UKPDS): clinical and therapeutic implications for type 2 diabetes. Br J Clin Pharmacol 1999;48(5):643–8.

5. Heller SR, The ADVANCE Collaborative Group. A summary of the ADVANCE trial. Diabetes Care 2009;32(Suppl 2):S357–61.

6. The Action to Control Cardiovascular Risk in Diabetes Study Group. Effects of intensive glucose lowering in type 2 diabetes. N Engl J Med 2008;358:2545–59.

7. VADT Study Group. Glucose control and vascular complications in Veterans with type 2 diabetes. N Engl J Med 2009;360:129–39.

8. Kulkarni K, Castle G, Gregory R, et al, Diabetes Care and Education Dietetic Practice Group. Nutrition practice guidelines for type 1 diabetes mellitus positively affect dietitian practices and patient outcomes. J Am Diet Assoc 1998;98:62–70.

9. Scavone G, Manto A, Pitocco D, et al. Effect of carbohydrate counting and medical nutritional therapy on glycaemic control in type 1 diabetic subjects: a pilot study. Diabet Med 2010;27:477–9.

10. Coppell KJ, Kataoka M, Williams SM, et al. Nutritional intervention in patients with type 2 diabetes who are hyperglycaemic despite optimised drug treatment—Lifestyle Over and Above Drugs in Diabetes (LOADD) study: randomised controlled trial. BMJ 2010;341:c3337.

11. James PA, Oparil S, Carter BL, et al. 2014 evidence-based guideline for the management of high blood pressure in adults: report from the panel members appointed to the eighth Joint National Committee (JNC 8). JAMA 2015;311(5):507–20.

12. Stone NJ, Robinson J, Lichtenstein AH, et al. ACC/AHA guideline on the treatment of blood cholesterol to reduce atherosclerotic cardiovascular risk in adults a report of the American College of Cardiology/American Heart Association task force on practice guidelines. Circulation 2013. http://dx.doi.org/10.1016/j.jacc.2013.11.002.

13. Cannon CP, Blazing MA, Giugliano RP, et al, IMPROVE-IT Investigators. Ezetimibe added to statin therapy after acute coronary syndromes. N Engl J Med 2015;372:2387–97.

14. Aspirin use to prevent cardiovascular disease and colorectal cancer: preventive medication. Rockville, MD: United States Preventive Task Force; 2016. Available at: http://www.uspreventiveservicestaskforce.org/Page/Document/UpdateSummaryFinal/aspirin-to-prevent-cardiovascular-disease-and-cancer?ds=1&s=aspirin. Accessed May 1, 2016.

15. Peters SA, Huxley RR, Woodward M. Diabetes as a risk factor for stroke in women compared with men: a systematic review and meta-analysis of 64 cohorts, including 775,385 individuals and 12,539 strokes. Lancet 2014;383:1973–80.

16. Centers for Disease Control and Prevention. Recommended adult immunization schedule for adults aged 19 years or older, by vaccine and age group. United States, 2016. Available at: http://www.cdc.gov/vaccines/schedules/hcp/imz/adult.html. Accessed April 8, 2016.

17. Colberg SR, Albright AL, Blissmer BJ, et al. Exercise and type 2 diabetes: American College of Sports Medicine and the American Diabetes Association joint position statement. Diabetes Care 2010;33(12):e147–67.

18. Dugan JA. Exercise recommendations for type 2 diabetes. JAAPA 2016;29(1):13–8.

19. Marwick TH, Hordern MD, Miller T, et al. Exercise training for type 2 diabetes mellitus: impact on cardiovascular risk: a scientific statement from the American Heart Association. Circulation 2009;119:3244–62.

20. Screening for coronary artery disease with electrocardiography. United States Preventative Services Task Force; 2013. Available at: http://www.uspreventiveservicestaskforce.org/uspstf/uspsacad.htm. Accessed May 1, 2016.

21. Collins MM, Corcoran P, Perry IJ. Anxiety and depression symptoms in patients with diabetes. Diabet Med 2009;26(2):153–61.

22. Welch GW, Jacobson AM, Polonsky WH. The problem areas in diabetes scale: an evaluation of its clinical utility. Diabetes Care 1997;20(5):760–6.

23. Polonsky WH, Fisher L, Earles J, et al. Assessing psychosocial distress in diabetes. Diabetes Care 2005;28(3):626–31.
24. Johnson ST, Al Sayay F, Mathe N, et al. The relationship of diabetes-related distress and depressive symptoms with physical activity and dietary behaviors in adults with type 2 diabetes: a cross-sectional study. J Diabetes Complications 2016. http://dx.doi.org/10.1016/j.jdiacomp.2016.02.019.
25. Which quit smoking medication is right for you? Available at: http://smokefree.gov/explore-medications. Accessed May 1, 2016.

Antihyperglycemic Medications

Overwhelmed with Too Many Options?

Karen Beer, PA-C, MSPAS, RD, LD, CDE

KEYWORDS

- Sulfonylurea • Biguanide • Thiazolidinedione (TZD)
- Dipeptidyl peptidase (DPP)-4 inhibitor
- Sodium glucose cotransporter (SGLT)-2 inhibitor
- Glucagon-like peptide (GLP)-1 receptor agonist • Basal insulin • Prandial insulin

KEY POINTS

- Metformin, along with diet and exercise, is the first-line treatment in newly diagnosed type 2 diabetes mellitus.
- Glucagon-like peptide (GLP)-1 receptor agonists, sodium glucose cotransporter (SGLT)-2 inhibitors, dipeptidyl peptidase (DPP)-4 inhibitors, and thiazolidinediones (TZDS) have been suggested as alternatives to metformin monotherapy.
- Patients with type 1 diabetes mellitus must be started on insulin, either multiple daily injection (MDI) or insulin pump therapy.
- Insulin is the most potent glucose-lowering agent. It has no dose ceiling and is effective in most patients. It is required for many patients with type 2 diabetes mellitus at some point in the course of their disease process.

INTRODUCTION

The number and types of medications available to treat diabetes grow each year. There are currently 9 classes of oral medications, 2 types of injectable medications, and a variety of insulins. Which medication to prescribe a patient with poorly controlled diabetes becomes more challenging as new medications enter the marketplace. Fortunately, 2 excellent resources exist. The American Diabetes Association (ADA) and the American Association of Clinical Endocrinologists (AACE) provide guidance for medication selection. The ADA publishes new guidelines annually: the *Standards of Medical Care*, which appear each year in the January issue of *Diabetes Care*. The AACE publishes the periodically updated type 2 algorithm, most recently published in the January 2016 issue of *Endocrine Practice*.

Oregon Medical Group, 974 Cabriole Court, Eugene, OR 97401, USA
E-mail address: kbeer@oregonmed.net

Physician Assist Clin 2 (2017) 25–38
http://dx.doi.org/10.1016/j.cpha.2016.08.005
2405-7991/17/© 2016 Elsevier Inc. All rights reserved.
physicianassistant.theclinics.com

Barriers to patient adherence to diabetic regimens include several factors that relate directly to the medications themselves: complexity, multiple daily dosing, cost, and side effects. Where possible, providers should collaboratively select medication regimens with patients to minimize these obstacles. In addition, providers should take into consideration efficacy, weight, comorbidities, risk of hypoglycemia, and patient preference. The goal is blood glucose reduction with minimal side effects, especially hypoglycemia.[1,2]

Severe hypoglycemia is strongly associated with a variety of adverse clinical outcomes, including vascular events and death. It is not known whether hypoglycemia is a cause of these events or a marker of vulnerability to such events. In the Action in Diabetes and Vascular Disease: Preterax and Diamicron MR Controlled Evaluation trial, risk factors for severe hypoglycemia were older age, longer duration of diabetes, higher creatinine levels, lower body mass index, lower cognitive function, use of 3 or more oral glucose-lowering medications, history of smoking or microvascular disease, and assignment to the intensive glucose control group.[3]

Metformin, diet, and exercise are considered first-line treatments for patients with newly diagnosed type 2 diabetes mellitus. After 3 months, if hemoglobin A_{1c} targets are not reached, additional medication(s) may be chosen from any of the following: sulfonylureas, TZDs, DPP-4 inhibitors, SGLT-2 inhibitors, GLP-1 receptor agonists, or basal insulin. Each new class of noninsulin medications, when added to metformin, lowers hemoglobin A_{1c} approximately 0.9% to 1.1%.[1] The AACE now considers GLP-1 receptor agonists, SGLT-2 inhibitors, DPP-4 inhibitors, α-glucosidase inhibitors, sulfonylureas, glinides, and TZDs as acceptable alternatives to metformin as initial therapy.[2]

Insulin is often the last medication to be added, but insulin initiation should not be delayed in patients who do not achieve glycemic targets. For patients with hemoglobin A_{1c} greater than 9.0% and symptoms (polyuria, polydipsia, and weight loss) at diagnosis, initial treatment with insulin is preferable.[1]

BIGUANIDE: METFORMIN

Metformin is the preferred initial pharmacologic agent for type 2 diabetes mellitus, unless contraindicated. Metformin activates AMP-kinase to reduce hepatic glucose production. It is safe, efficacious, and inexpensive; promotes modest weight loss; and may lower risk of cardiovascular events and death.[1,2] Advantages of metformin include low cost, a long safety profile, absence of hypoglycemia and, based on results of the United Kingdom Prospective Diabetes Study (UKPDS), reduction in cardiovascular events.[1,2,4] Disadvantages of metformin include gastrointestinal side effects (diarrhea, nausea/vomiting, and flatulence), vitamin B_{12}, deficiency, and a low risk of lactic acidosis. Vitamin B_{12} levels should be monitored in patients on this medication and supplements advised when deficiency is identified.[2] Contraindications to use of metformin include chronic kidney disease, acidosis, hypoxia, and dehydration.[1]

Metformin should be started at 500 mg, once or twice per day with meals, and titrated by 500 mg weekly to 1000 mg twice per day with meals to minimize gastrointestinal side effects. Gastrointestinal side effects may limit maximal dosing.[5] If gastrointestinal side effects appear, patients may revert to the highest previously tolerated dose. Modestly greater effectiveness is seen at doses up to 2500 mg/d. Metformin has been shown to lower hemoglobin A_{1c} approximately 1% compared with placebo after 3 months. Gastrointestinal side effects may be lessened by using extended release products.

Metformin may be safely continued to a glomerular filtration rate (GFR) of 45 mL/min or even 30 mL/min. When used in patients with GFR in the lower range, the dose should be lowered and patients advised to stop it in the event of nausea, vomiting, or dehydration. Metformin should also be stopped prior to administration of radiocontrast dye in those with estimated GFR (eGFR) less than 60 mL/min.[1,2,6]

Metformin should be continued as background therapy as other agents are added. Metformin plus a second agent should be started on patients who present with hemoglobin A$_{1c}$ greater than 7.5%. Consider 2 medications with complementary mechanisms of actions.[2]

A meta-analysis showed that metformin, when used in overweight or obese patients with type 1 diabetes mellitus, reduced insulin requirements, body weight, and total and low-density lipoprotein cholesterol (LDL-C) but did not significantly lower hemoglobin A$_{1c}$.[7]

INSULIN SECRETAGOGUES: SULFONYLUREAS AND MEGLITINIDES

Secretagogues close the potassium-ATP channels on the plasma membrane of beta cells, resulting in increased insulin secretion.

Sulfonylureas

The sulfonylureas are glyburide, glipizide, and glimepiride. They should be taken with meals. Advantages of sulfonylureas include low cost, long history of use, and, based on results of the UKPDS,[4] decreased microvascular risk. Disadvantages are their propensity for hypoglycemia and weight gain.[1,4] Outside of insulin, sulfonylureas have the highest risk of serious hypoglycemia. They are potent but lack durability.[2] Sulfonylureas demonstrate hemoglobin A$_{1c}$ lowering of 1.25%.[8]

Sulfonylureas may be discontinued when mealtime insulin is started, given the similar mechanisms of action. When sulfonylureas are used in combination with insulin, the risks of hypoglycemia and weight gain increase.[2]

Meglitinides

Meglitinides, rapid-acting secretagogues, are useful when the goal is to reduce postprandial blood glucose spikes. These medications are repaglinide and nateglinide. They are taken with carbohydrate-containing meals and should be omitted when meals are skipped. They can result in hypoglycemia and weight gain.[1,2] They have shorter half-lives, a lower hemoglobin A$_{1c}$–lowering effect, and lower risk of hypoglycemia than sulfonylureas.[2] They lower hemoglobin A$_{1c}$ by approximately 0.75%.[8]

THIAZOLIDINEDIONES

The TZDs, pioglitazone and rosiglitazone, activate nuclear transcription factor peroxisome proliferator-activated receptor-γ to enhance insulin sensitivity. They are inexpensive, offer durability, do not cause hypoglycemia, and raise high-density lipoprotein cholesterol.[1,2] Pioglitazone lowers triglycerides, and, according to results of the PROspective pioglitAzone Clinical Trial In macroVascular Events, also reduces cardiovascular events.[9] TZDs lower hemoglobin A$_{1c}$ by 1% to 1.25%.[8]

Adverse effects include the potential for weight gain, edema, heart failure, and bone fracture.[1,2] Rosiglitazone has been shown to raise LDL-C and, in a 2007 meta-analysis by Nissen, showed increased risk of myocardial infarction and cardiovascular death.[1,10] But reanalysis of this data demonstrated no increased risk and led to the reversal of all restrictions.[11] Revised labeling reflects the altered view of rosiglitazone and currently states only that rosiglitazone may be used to help control blood sugar in type 2 diabetes mellitus. GlaxoSmithKline, was also released from postmarketing requirements to conduct the Thiazolidinedione Intervention with Vitamin D Evaluation trial comparing rosiglitazone to pioglitazone and other diabetes drugs, stating that it had "concluded that this trial is no longer necessary or feasible."

Pioglitazone may be used with insulin at doses of 15 mg and 30 mg but may aggravate weight gain.[2]

In the Insulin Resistance Intervention after Stroke study, pioglitazone was used in patients with insulin resistance, but not diabetes, and a recent ischemic stroke or transient ischemic attack. It reduced the risk of fatal or nonfatal stroke or myocardial infarct by 24%, from 11.8% to 9%, after less than 5 years of treatment compared with patients treated with placebo.[12]

INCRETIN MIMETICS: DIPEPTIDYL PEPTIDASE 4 INHIBITORS AND GLUCAGON-LIKE PEPTIDE 1 AGONISTS

Incretins (GLP-1 and gastric inhibitory polypeptide) stimulate beta cells to produce more insulin in a glucose-dependent way. They also suppress alpha cells from producing glucagon, which lowers hepatogluconeogenesis. Incretins slow gastric emptying and enhance satiety.[1,2]

Dipeptidyl Peptidase 4 Inhibitors

DPP-4 is the enzyme that deactivates incretins; by inhibiting this enzyme, incretin action is prolonged. Sitagliptin, saxagliptin, linagliptin, and alogliptin are the currently available DPP-4 inhibitors. DPP-4 inhibitors are well tolerated and do not cause hypoglycemia. They have modest hemoglobin A_{1c}–lowering capability and are weight neutral. DPP-4 inhibitors lower hemoglobin A_{1c} approximately 0.75% versus placebo.[8]

The DPP-4 inhibitors can cause angioedema, urticaria other immune-mediated dermatologic effects and severe and persistent joint pain; may be implicated in acute pancreatitis; and are expensive.[1,2,13]

Except for linagliptin, the DPP-4 inhibitors are renally excreted; therefore, doses should be adjusted for renal impairment.

In March 2016, the Food and Drug Administration (FDA) submitted a safety alert for saxagliptin and alogliptin, highlighting 2 large clinical trials conducted in patients with heart disease that showed more patients who received saxagliptin or alogliptin were hospitalized for heart failure compared with patients receiving placebo. Risk factors included a history of heart failure or renal impairment. These medications should be stopped in patients who develop heart failure.[14]

Glucagon-Like Peptide 1 Receptor Agonists

Exenatide, exenatide extended release, liraglutide, albiglutide, and dulaglutide are GLP-1 receptor agonists. They activate GLP-1 receptors, resulting in increased glucose-dependent insulin secretion, decreased glucagon secretion, slowed gastric emptying, and increased satiety. They are more powerful than the DPP-4 inhibitors and decrease both fasting and postprandial glucose.[1,2] Hemoglobin A_{1c} lowering varies from 0.87% to 1.9% with a low risk of hypoglycemia. GLP-1 receptor agonists reduce blood pressure and other cardiovascular risk factors and are useful when weight loss is desired. Weight loss over 3 to 4 months of treatment is 1.4 kg to 3.87 kg.[15]

Disadvantages of the GLP-1 receptor agonists include gastrointestinal side effects (nausea, vomiting, and diarrhea), increased heart rate, injectable administration and the need for patient training.[1,2] Nausea is generally transient and resolves with continued treatment.[15]

Some GLP-1 agonists are administered once a week, whereas others are administered daily or even twice a day. A meta-analysis comparing the efficacy of the once-weekly GLP-1 agonists showed the greatest reduction in hemoglobin A_{1c}, fasting plasma glucose, and body weight with dulaglutide, followed by once-weekly exenatide.[16]

GLP-1 agonists are contraindicated in patients with personal or family history of medullary thyroid cancer or multiple endocrine neoplasia syndrome type 2. They may be implicated in acute pancreatitis.[1,2] Exenatide should not be used if creatinine clearance is less than 30 mL/min. Because of their effect on gastric emptying, use in patients with gastroparesis requires careful monitoring.[2]

Consider adding a GLP-1 agonist when patients on maximal monotherapy or dual therapy are unable to achieve hemoglobin A_{1c} targets. When a GLP-1 is added to insulin, insulin doses may need to be decreased to avoid hypoglycemia.

AMYLIN MIMETICS

Pramlintide is the only available amylin mimetic. It is FDA approved for both type 1 diabetes mellitus and type 2 diabetes mellitus and with MDI regimens.[1,2] It activates amylin receptors to decrease glucagon secretion, slow gastric emptying, and improve satiety. Advantages include reduced postprandial glucose excursion and weight loss. Disadvantages include modest hemoglobin A_{1c} lowering and gastrointestinal side effects, such as nausea and vomiting. It can cause hypoglycemia if insulin doses are not simultaneously reduced. Pramlintide is injectable, must be dosed frequently, requires patient training, and is expensive.[1]

SODIUM GLUCOSE COTRANSPORTER 2 INHIBITORS

SGLT-2 inhibitors include canagliflozin, dapagliflozin, and empagliflozin. They inhibit the action of glucose transporters in the proximal nephron, to decrease renal glucose reabsorption, and thereby increase glycosuria. SGLT-2 inhibitors offer the advantages of no hypoglycemia, weight loss, blood pressure reduction, and efficacy at all stages of type 2 diabetes mellitus.[1,2] In the Empagliflozin, Cardiovascular Outcomes, and Mortality in Type 2 Diabetes trial, empagliflozin was associated with lower risk of death from cardiovascular causes, death from any cause and hospitalization for heart failure in patients with type 2 diabetes mellitus, and cardiovascular disease compared with placebo.[17]

Disadvantages of SGLT-2 inhibitors include genitourinary infections, polyuria, volume depletion, hypotension, dizziness, LDL-C elevation, transient creatinine elevation, diabetic ketoacidosis (DKA), urosepsis, and pyelonephritis.[1,2] Dose reductions may be required for eGFR less than 60 mL/min, and they have limited efficacy in patients with eGFR less than 45 mL/min.[2,17]

Postmarket reports have implicated SGLT-2 inhibitors in euglycemic DKA, and investigations are ongoing. In some affected patients, a precipitant, such as major illness, reduced food or fluid intake, or reduced insulin dose, may have triggered the event, and some were subsequently diagnosed as having autoimmune (type 1) diabetes mellitus. Patients started on these medications should be warned to avoid dehydration and to be alert to symptoms of potential DKA, including nausea, vomiting, abdominal pain, fatigue, or dyspnea.[2,18,19] An AACE/American College of Endocrinology expert consensus panel performed a thorough review and recommended no changes to SGLT-2 inhibitor labeling, but in December 2015, the FDA revised

SGLT-2 inhibitors labeling to include warnings about euglycemic DKA and serious urinary tract infections.[2,18]

In April 2016, the European Medicines Agency announced it was reviewing canagliflozin after results of a trial, the Canagliflozin Cardiovascular Assessment Study, showed a slight increase in lower extremity amputation in the canagliflozin-treated population.[20]

Although the SGLT-2 inhibitors have been studied in type 1 diabetes mellitus, they are currently only FDA approved for use in type 2 diabetes mellitus.[21]

BILE ACID SEQUESTRANTS

Colesevelam binds bile acids in the intestinal tract, to increase bile acid excretion in the stool. It decreases the amount of bile acids returned to the liver, thereby increasing hepatic bile acid production. Its mechanism of action is incompletely understood, but it may decrease hepatic glucose production and increase incretin levels. It does not cause hypoglycemia and lowers LDL-C. It can cause constipation and dyspepsia, raise triglycerides, and decrease absorption of other medications. For these reasons, its modest effect on hemoglobin A_{1c} lowering and its high cost, it is infrequently prescribed.[1,2]

DOPAMINE AGONISTS

Bromocriptine has been used for years for prolactinoma and Parkinson disease; it has been reformulated as a quick-release product to be taken early in the morning for diabetes. Quick-release bromocriptine activates dopaminergic receptors to modulate hypothalamic regulation of metabolism and increase insulin sensitivity. Advantages include absence of hypoglycemia and reduced cardiovascular events, seen in the Cycloset Safety Trial.[22] But its modest hemoglobin A_{1c}-lowering, side effects (which include dizziness syncope, nausea, fatigue, and rhinitis) and high cost, make it a less desirable option.[1,2] It should not be used in patients taking antipsychotic medications.[2]

α-GLUCOSIDASE INHIBITORS

The α-glucosidase inhibitors, acarbose and miglitol, inhibit intestinal α-glucosidase, an enzyme located on the intestinal brush border. This enzyme breaks down starches and disaccharides to glucose. These medications slow intestinal carbohydrate digestion and absorption. They act locally to reduce postprandial glucose excursions without hypoglycemia. The Study to Prevent Non-Insulin-Dependent Diabetes Mellitus demonstrated their ability to lower blood pressure and decrease cardiovascular events.[23] They offer modest hemoglobin A_{1c} lowering if taken with all carbohydrate-containing meals. They cause bloating, flatulence, and diarrhea and should be used in caution in patients with renal impairment.[1,2]

INSULIN

Insulin is the most potent glucose-lowering agent. Insulin activates insulin receptors to increase glucose disposal, decrease hepatic glucose production, and suppress ketogenesis.[2] Patients respond nearly universally, efficacy is theoretically unlimited, and results of the UKPDS demonstrate microvascular risk lowering.[1,2,4] Insulin causes hypoglycemia and weight gain and may have mitogenic effects.[1]

Patients and providers are often reluctant to start insulin, but its use should not be seen as failure or punishment, because the progressive nature of diabetes leads many patients with type 2 diabetes mellitus to require it at some point in their disease process. Insulin must be injected or (in the case of prandial insulin) inhaled. Patients must be trained to administer it, and it can be expensive.[1]

Insulin pharmacokinetics and pharmacodynamics are affected by injection site. Heat and muscle activity increase insulin absorption rate. Insulin action can also be affected by massage, bathing in warm water, and vasodilating or vasoconstricting medications.[24] Insulin doses, particularly of rapid-acting insulin, prior to or just after any of these activities may need to be reduced to avoid hypoglycemia.

Abdominal subcutaneous tissue provides more predictable absorption than the thigh or deltoid, because it is not as prone to the effects of heat, exercise, and activity as muscle. Insulin injection site rotation within a single location each week is recommended to decrease variability and improve predictability of insulin response.[24]

Thirty to 80% of circulating insulin is cleared by the kidney; therefore, insulin clearance is decreased in the elderly and those with renal dysfunction. Frequent blood glucose testing and insulin dose reduction are recommended in these populations to reduce risk of hypoglycemia.[24]

Severely obese patients may require larger doses and split doses to improve insulin action and predictability.[24]

Insulin has traditionally been administered using vial and syringe. Virtually all insulins, however, are available in pen form. The pen offers convenience and is simpler to manage, particularly when patients have decreased vision or dexterity challenges.[25] Insulin pens may be more expensive than vials. It is important for providers to remember to prescribe pen needles or syringes along with insulin pen devices or vials.

Basal Insulins

Glargine, detemir, and degludec are the currently available basal insulin analogs. All have onsets of 1 hour. Glargine and detemir have durations of approximately 24 hours.[26] Their relatively flat profiles reduce risk of hypoglycemia.[24,27,28] Detemir and glargine differ slightly in their pharmacodynamics and pharmacokinetics. Small doses may result in a shorter half-life, and users may find flatter time-action profiles with twice-daily dosing, especially with detemir.[24,25,29] With larger doses, area under the curve and duration of action are increased.[24]

Glargine and detemir may be given any time of the day, as long as they are given at the same time each day. In studies, glargine has traditionally been given at bedtime,[30] but some patients may find it easier to remember first thing in the morning.

Due to its lower pH, glargine, when given via syringe, may not be mixed with other insulins. The acidic solution may sting or burn when injected.

Patients may be instructed on administration and told to inject a single bedtime dose, such as 10 U or 0.1 U/kg to 0.2 U/kg, depending on the degree of hyperglycemia, with instructions for self-titration until a desirable fasting glucose is reached.[1]

Degludec has a duration of 42 hours.[28] It has demonstrated less variability and more stability in maintaining glycemic control compared with glargine when studied in patients with type 1 diabetes mellitus. It was as effective as glargine whether given once daily or 3 times a week in patients with type 2 diabetes mellitus.[31] Longer duration of action allows for greater flexibility in dosing. This may be useful when schedules are variable or unpredictable, for example, in cases of shift workers who switch from day shift to night shift.

When basal insulin alone does not provide adequate glycemic control, consider adding a GLP-1 receptor agonist, an SGLT-2 inhibitor, or a DPP-4 inhibitor. These medications, when added to insulin, limit postprandial blood glucose excursion, weight gain, and risk of hypoglycemia. In these instances, insulin dose reduction may be required to prevent hypoglycemia.[2]

Intermediate-Acting Insulin

Intermediate-acting insulin (NPH insulin) may be used as a basal insulin at much lower cost than basal insulin analogs.[1] It is equally effective at hemoglobin A_{1c} lowering, but it is more likely to cause hypoglycemia than basal insulin analogs and should be avoided in patients with a history of nocturnal hypoglycemia.[2,30,32] Limitations include a pronounced peak, limited duration, and erratic absorption.[27] NPH insulin has an onset of 1 to 3 hours, peaks at 6 to 8 hours, and lasts 12 to 16 hours.[26,33]

NPH insulin has been used effectively to deal with steroid-induced hyperglycemia, because its action profile closely matches the pattern of hyperglycemia seen in patients treated with prednisone and methylprednisolone. In these cases, it is given once a day in the morning, and doses are titrated based on steroid dose and blood glucose.[34,35]

Rapid-Acting Insulin Analogs

If basal insulin titrated to a target fasting blood glucose still does not result in hemoglobin A_{1c} at goal, rapid-acting insulin may be added at 1 or more meals per day to control postprandial glucose excursions.[1,2]

Rapid-acting insulin analogs (insulin lispro, insulin aspart, and insulin glulisine) and inhaled insulin activate insulin receptors to increase glucose disposal and reduce hepatic glucose production in the postprandial state. In contrast to basal insulins, they have a prompt onset of action and lend themselves to administration immediately prior to meals. Rapid-acting insulins have an onset of 15 minutes, a peak at 30 to 90 minutes, and duration of 3 to 5 hours.[1,2,26]

Insulin analogs are preferable to human insulins due to their more rapid action and decreased hypoglycemia. Ideally, insulin doses should be matched to carbohydrate intake, premeal blood glucose, and anticipated physical activity.[1,2]

Inhaled Insulin

Inhaled insulin is available for prandial use only. It may be an option for those with needle phobia, but it has a limited dosing range and should be started only after spirometry is used to rule out existing lung problems.[36] Additionally, lung function should be monitored periodically with spirometer in patients treated with inhaled insulin. It should not be used in active smokers or patients with asthma or chronic obstructive pulmonary disease. Inhaled insulin demonstrates inferior hemoglobin A_{1c} lowering compared with rapid-acting insulin.[1] It is available in single-use cartridges of 4 U, 8 U, and 12 U,[36] making strict adherence to an insulin-to-carbohydrate ratio (ICR) challenging.

Short-Acting Insulin

Regular insulin was the only prandial insulin available prior to the advent of insulin analogs. U-100 regular insulin, also referred to as short-acting insulin, has an onset of 30 to 60 minutes, a peak at 2 to 4 hours, and duration of 5 to 8 hours.[26,33] This increase in plasma insulin levels long after meals can increase risk of postprandial hypoglycemia.[24] It should be taken 30 minutes prior to the start of meals.

It may be useful in patients with gastroparesis and may be a consideration when cost of rapid-acting insulin analogs is prohibitive.[24] It is available in pen and vial.

Premixed Insulins

Premixed insulins include 70/30 NPH insulin and regular insulin, 70/30 NPH insulin and insulin aspart, 75/25 NPH insulin and insulin lispro, and 50/50 NPH insulin and regular insulin. Premixed insulins offer less frequent dosing but provide less flexibility and require a rigid eating schedule. They are associated with an increased frequency of hypoglycemia.[2]

IDegAsp is a combined basal/rapid-acting insulin.[28] It is expected to be available in 70%/30% and 55%/45% formulations.[31]

Concentrated Insulins

For patients with significant insulin resistance and high insulin demands, several options exist. Insulin glargine U-300 and insulin degludec U-200 are basal insulins that are 3 and 2 times more concentrated, respectively, than glargine U-100 and degludec U-100.[1] Individuals with insulin resistance may require 2 U/kg or more.[25] Given these high doses, concentrated insulins may be better absorbed due to a smaller volume.

The rate of nocturnal hypoglycemia is reduced with degludec U-200 and glargine U-300 compared with U-100 glargine.[25] Other benefits include decreased volume of administered insulin, reduced injection burden and flexible administration timing.

Studies demonstrate the glucose-lowering effect of glargine U-300 lasts more than 30 hours.[25] Degludec U-200 like degludec U-100 lasts 42 hours.[25,28] Glargine U-300 like glargine U-100 should not be mixed with other insulins due to its low pH.

U-500 regular insulin is 5 times more concentrated per volume than U-100, providing 500 U of insulin in 1 mL of solution. Available since the 1950s, it is approved for use in type 1 diabetes mellitus and type 2 diabetes mellitus. It has been studied in pregnancy and has category B listing. It is indicated individuals using greater than 200 U/d of insulin.[25] It has recently become available in a pen device.

It has a similar onset but longer duration of action than U-100 regular insulin. U-500 regular insulin peaks at approximately 30 minutes; insulin action lasts approximately 7 hours.[25] This delayed effect allows it to be used for both basal and prandial coverage. It should be given 30 minutes prior to meals.

U-500 regular insulin has been studied in patients using both MDI regimens and insulin pump therapy and has demonstrated the capability to lower hemoglobin A_{1c} in obese patients. These studies also report weight gain and an increase in the number of insulin units used. Adherence may be improved given the potential to reduce injection burden from 5 to 6 shots per day to 2 or 3 shots per day with U-500. There may be a small increase in hypoglycemia seen with transition to the use of U-500 regular insulin.[25]

Two different algorithms for dosing U-500 in insulin resistant patients were compared. Patients with uncontrolled type 2 diabetes mellitus taking more than 200 U/d of U-100 insulin were randomized to either 2 shots per day or 3 shots per day of U-500 regular insulin. Total daily insulin doses were reduced by 20% in patients with hemoglobin A_{1c} less than or equal to 8% or average self-monitored plasma glucose (SMPG) less than 183 md/dL. Otherwise, patients were started on U-500 insulin at the same total daily dose (TDD) as U-100 insulin. Doses were given at breakfast, lunch, and dinner for the 3-times-a-day group and at breakfast and dinner for the twice-a-day group. Insulin distribution was either 40%/30%/30% or 60%/40%. Doses were adjusted up by 5% to 15% for hyperglycemia or down by 5% for hypoglycemia to a target premeal SMPG of 71 mg/dL to 130 mg/dL. Hemoglobin A_{1c} lowering of 1.12% was seen in the 3-times-a-day group and 1.22% in the twice-a-day group; 15% and 17% of the 3-times-a-day and twice-a-day groups, respectively, reached a hemoglobin A_{1c} of 6.5% or less; 29% and 31% of the 3-times-a-day and twice-a-day groups, respectively, reached a hemoglobin A_{1c} of less than 7%. Insulin doses, hypoglycemia, and weight gain were similar between groups.[37]

One rapid-acting insulin, insulin lispro, is also available in concentrated form. Insulin lispro U-200 is recommended when prandial doses are sizable.

INITIATION AND ADJUSTMENT OF INSULIN REGIMENS

Insulin should be started in patients with type 2 diabetes mellitus and symptoms, significantly elevated blood glucoses and/or hemoglobin A_{1c} greater than 9.0%. Insulin doses may be reduced as glucose levels improve.[1,2] Insulin should be considered in patients with long-standing type 2 diabetes mellitus on 2 oral agents and hemoglobin A_{1c} greater than 8.0%.[2]

Insulin regimens should be designed with lifestyle and mealtimes in mind. The simplest way to introduce insulin is with a single daily dose of basal insulin.[2] A once-daily basal insulin may be started at 10 U/kg or 0.2 U/kg. Dose adjustment should be done on a frequent and regular basis based on fasting blood glucose, either by a health care professional or a trained patient. Patients may be instructed on dose titration based on a fasting blood glucose target.[2,5,30,32] For example, patients may be instructed to increase the dose by 2 U every 3 days until fasting levels are consistently 70 mg/dL to 130 mg/dL. If fasting glucoses are 180 or higher, doses may be increased more rapidly, for example, by 4 U every 3 days. If hypoglycemia occurs, or the fasting glucose drops below 70 mg/dL, reduce the basal insulin by 4 U or 10%, whichever is greater.[5]

After 2 or 3 months, if hemoglobin A_{1c} is 7% or greater, add rapid-acting insulin based on the results of premeal blood glucoses. Prandial insulin may be given for 1 meal per day or may be given at all 3 meals. Begin with 4 U of a rapid-acting insulin at the start of the meal, and increase by 2 U every 3 days until blood glucose at the following meal is in range. For example, if prelunch blood glucose is out of range, give rapid-acting insulin at breakfast. If bedtime glucose is out of range, add rapid-acting insulin at dinner, and so forth.[5]

After 3 months, if hemoglobin A_{1c} continues to be out of range, patients may be instructed to check 2-hour postprandial blood glucose levels and adjust preprandial rapid acting insulin doses accordingly.[5] The ADA recommends a peak postprandial (1–2 hours) blood glucose less than 180,[38] whereas AACE recommends 2-hour postprandial blood glucose goal less than 140 mg/dL.[2]

MDI therapy, or pairing basal insulin with prandial and correction doses, should be started in patients with blood glucoses 300 mg/dL or higher, a hemoglobin A_{1c} of 10% or higher, or when catabolic features, such as weight loss or ketosis, are present. Regimens may be simplified as glucose toxicity resolves.[1]

For patients with type 1 diabetes mellitus, insulin is the mainstay of therapy.[1] Either MDIs or subcutaneous continuous insulin infusion, also known as insulin pump therapy, is appropriate. Increasing insurance reimbursement has allowed more and more patients with type 2 diabetes mellitus to use insulin pumps.

Both MDI and subcutaneous continuous insulin infusion can be maximized through the use of ICRs and insulin sensitivity factors (ISFs). These formulas help educated patients more closely estimate the appropriate dose of rapid-acting insulin to administer when the current SMPG and the amount of carbohydrates (in grams) to be consumed are known. These can be calculated by the provider using formulas. Such formulas have been developed for patients with type 1 diabetes mellitus but may be extrapolated for use in patients with type 2 mellitus.

The ICR is defined as the number of grams of carbohydrate that are covered by a single unit of bolus insulin. Commonly used formulas are 400/TDD or 500/TDD, where TDD equals the average total daily (basal and rapid-acting insulin combined) insulin used.

Table 1 Formulas	
	Example
Calculating ICR and ISF	Basal dose: 25 U Prandial dose: 6–8 U 3 times a day with each meal TDD: ~50 U *ICR*: 500/TDD → 500/50 → *10* *ISF*: 1700/TDD → 1700/50 → *34*
Calculating dose	Patient premeal glucose is 168 and plans to eat 40 g of CHO Insulin for meal: consuming CHO/ICR → 40/10 → *4* U Insulin for correction: (premeal glucose – target glucose)/ISF → (168–100)/34 → 68/34 → *2* U
Dose to administer	Insulin for meal + insulin for correction → 4 + 2 → *6* U

ISF (commonly referred as "correction factor") is defined as the number of points (mg/dL) blood glucose is expected to decrease in response to administration of 1 U of rapid- or short-acting. The often-used formula for calculating insulin sensitivity is 1700/TDD.[37,38] The number of units to be taken for a high blood glucose, then, is (target blood glucose minus actual blood glucose) divided by ISF. The premeal insulin dose is the sum of the carbohydrate dose and the high blood glucose (correction) dose (**Table 1**).

These formulas have been analyzed and criticized. More accurate formulas have been published,[39,40] but they are more complex and may be less likely to be used by a busy clinician. These formulas serve as a starting place for patients to begin insulin dose self-adjustment and can be modified as needed based on blood glucose records at subsequent office visits. Insulin pumps (and other diabetes regimens, including MDI) are now sometimes paired with continuous glucose monitors, which check and communicate the blood glucose using interstitial fluid every 5 minutes. Continuous glucose monitors alert the wearer to threshold lows or highs, and can, when paired with insulin pumps, trigger the insulin pump to suspend insulin delivery to arrest nocturnal hypoglycemia.[1]

SUMMARY

Selecting the most appropriate medication for a patient with diabetes can be confusing, given the ever-expanding list of available medications. Medication selection should take into consideration efficacy, cost, adverse drug effects, weight, comorbidities, risk of hypoglycemia and patient preference. The goal is blood glucose reduction with minimal side effects, especially hypoglycemia. Hypoglycemia is dangerous and may be a deterrent to medication adherence. Patients may fail to adhere to diabetic regimens for a variety of reasons, including complexity, multiple daily dosing, cost, and side effects. It behooves providers to work with patients to select medication regimens that patients are likely to follow.

Metformin, diet, and exercise are the recommended initial treatments for patients with newly diagnosed type 2 diabetes mellitus. The AACE now considers GLP-1 receptor agonists, SGLT-2 inhibitors, DPP-4 inhibitors, α-glucosidase inhibitors, sulfonylureas, glinides, and TZDs as acceptable alternatives to metformin as initial therapy. Additional medications may be chosen when hemoglobin A_{1c} targets are not met. Insulin should be prescribed for patients with hemoglobin A_{1c} greater than 9.0% and symptoms at diagnosis.

REFERENCES

1. American Diabetes Association. Approaches to glycemic treatment. Sec. 7. In Standards of Medical Care in Diabetes—2016. Diabetes Care 2016;39(Suppl 1):S52–9.
2. Garber AJ, Abrahamson MJ, Barzilay JI, et al. AACE/ACE consensus statement: consensus statement by the American Association of Clinical Endocrinologist and American College of Endocrinology on the comprehensive type 2 diabetes management algorithm.—2016 executive summary. Endocr Pract 2016;22(10): 84–113.
3. Zoungas S, Patel A, Chalmers J, et al. Severe hypoglycemia and risks of vascular events and death. N Engl J Med 2010;363(15):1410–8.
4. UKPDS Study Group. UK prospective study of therapies of maturity-onset diabetes. I. Effect of diet, sulphonylurea, insulin or biguanide therapy on fasting plasma glucose and body weight over one year. Diabetologia 1983;24:404–11.
5. Nathan DM, Buse JB, Davison MB, et al. Medical management of hyperglycemia in type 2 diabetes: a consensus algorithm for the initiation and adjustment of therapy: a consensus statement of the American Diabetes Association and the European Association for the Study of Diabetes. Diabetes Care 2009;32(1):193–203.
6. American Diabetes Association. Microvascular complications and foot care. Sec 9. In Standards of Medical Care in Diabetes—2016. Diabetes Care 2016; 39(Suppl 1):S72–80.
7. Vella S, Buetow L, Royle P, et al. The use of metformin in type 1 diabetes: a systematic review of efficacy. Diabetologia 2010;53(5):809–20.
8. Sherifali D, Nerenberg K, Pullenayegum E, et al. The effect of oral antidiabetic agents of A1c levels. Diabetes Care 2010;33(8):1859–64.
9. Dormandy JA, Charbonnel B, Eckland DJA, et al, on behalf of the PROactive Investigators. Secondary prevention of macrovascular events in patients with type 2 diabetes in the PROactive Study (PROspective pioglitAzone Clinical Trial In macroVascular Events): a randomised controlled trial. Lancet 2005;366:1279–89.
10. Nissen SE, Wolski K. Effect of rosiglitazone on the risk of myocardial infarction and death from cardiovascular causes. N Engl J Med 2008;356:2457–71.
11. Husten L. FDA removes restrictions on Avandia. Forbes 2013. Accessed June 9, 2016.
12. Kernan WN, Viscoli KL, Fuiri LH, et al. Pioglitazone after ischemic stroke or transient ischemic attack. N Engl J Med 2016;374(14):1321–31.
13. US Food and Drug Administration. Drug safety communication: FDA warns that DPP-4 inhibitors for type 2 diabetes may cause severe joint pain. Available at: http://www.fda.gov/safety/medwatch/safetyinformation/safetyalertsforhumanmedicalproducts/ucm494252.htm. Accessed April 29, 2016.
14. US Food and Drug Administration. Drug safety communication: diabetes medication containing saxagliptin and alogliptin– risk of heart failure. Available at: http://www.fda.gov/safety/medwatch/safetyinformation/safetyalertsforhumanmedicalproducts/ucm494252.htm. Accessed April 14, 2016.
15. Garber AJ. Long-acting glucagon-like peptide 1 receptor agonists. Diabetes Care 2011;34(S2):S279–84.
16. Zaccardi F, Htike ZZ, Webb DR, et al. Benefits and harms of once-weekly glucagon-like peptide-1 receptor agonist treatments: a systematic review and network meta-analysis. Ann Intern Med 2016;164(2):102–13.
17. Zinman B, Wanner C, Lachin JM, et al. Empagliflozin, cardiovascular outcomes, and mortality in type 2 diabetes. N Engl J Med 2015;373(22):2117–27.

18. US Food and Drug Administration. FDA drug safety communication: FDA warns that SGLT2 inhibitors for diabetes may result in a serious condition of too much acid in the blood. [article online]. 2015. Available at: http://www.fda.gov/Drugs/DrugSafety/ucm446845.htm. Accessed April 23, 2016.
19. Erondu N, Desai M, Ways K, et al. Diabetes ketoacidosis and related events in the canagliflozin type 2 diabetes clinical program. Diabetes Care 2015;38:1680–6.
20. European Medicines Agency. EMA reviews diabetes medicine canagliflozin. London. 2016. EMA/267042/2016. Accessed April 23, 2016.
21. Perkins BA, Cherney DZI, Partridge H, et al. Sodium-glucose cotransporter 2 inhibition and glycemic control in type 1 diabetes; results of an 8-week open-label proof-of-concept trial. Diabetes Care 2014;37:1480–3.
22. Gaziano JM, Cincotta AH, O'Connor CM, et al. Randomized clinical trial of quick-release bromocriptine among patient with type 2 diabetes on overall safety and cardiovascular outcomes. Diabetes Care 2010;33(7):1503–8.
23. Chiasson JL, Josse RG, Gomis R, et al. Acarbose treatment and the risk of cardiovascular disease and hypertension in patients with impaired glucose tolerance: the STOP-NIDDM Trial. JAMA 2003;290(4):486–94.
24. Morello CM. Pharmacokinetics and pharmacodynamics of insulin analogs in special populations with type 2 diabetes mellitus. Int J Gen Med 2011;4:827–35.
25. Lamos EM, Younk LM, Davis SN. Concentrated insulins: the new basal insulins. Ther Clin Risk Manag 2016;12:389–400.
26. National Institutes of Health: National Institute of Diabetes and Digestive and Kidney Diseases. Insert C: types of insulin. In What I need to know about Diabetes Medicines. Available at: http://www.niddk.nih.gov/health-information/health-topics/Diabetes/diabetes-medicines/Pages/insert_C.aspx. Accessed April 17, 2016.
27. Heise T, Pieber TR. Toward peakless, reproducible and long-acting insulin. An assessment of the basal analogues based on isoglycaemic clamp studies. Diabetes Obes Metab 2007;9:648–59.
28. Kalra S. Basal insulin analogues in the treatment of diabetes mellitus: what progress have we made? Indian J Endocrinol Metab 2015;19(Suppl 1):S71–3.
29. Porcellati F, Bolli GB, Fanelli CG. Pharmacokinetics and pharmacodynamics of basal insulins. Diabetes Technol Ther 2011;13(Suppl 1):S15–24.
30. Riddle MC, Rosenstock J, Gerich J. The treat-to-target trial: randomized addition of glargine or human NPH insulin to oral therapy of type 2 diabetes. Diabetes Care 2003;26(11):3080–6.
31. Kalra S, Unnikrishnan A, Baruah M, et al. Degludec insulin: a novel basal insulin. Indian J Endocrinol Metab 2011;15(Suppl 1):S12–6.
32. Hermansen K, Davies M, Derezinski T, et al. A 26-week, randomized, parallel, treat-to-target trial comparing insulin determir with NPH insulin as add-on therapy to oral glucose lowering drugs in insulin-naïve people with type 2 diabetes. Diabetes Care 2006;26(6):1269–74.
33. Woodworth JR, Howey DC, Bowsher RR. Establishment of time-action profiles for regular and NPH insulin using pharmacodynamic modeling. Diabetes Care 1994;17(1):64–9.
34. Seggelke SA, Gibbs J, Draznin B. Pilot study of using neutral protamine hagedorn insulin to counteract the effect of methylprednisolone in hospitalized patients with diabetes. J Hosp Med 2011;6:175–6.
35. Grommesh B, Lausch MJ, Vannelli AJ, et al. Hospital insulin protocol aims for glucose control in glucocorticoid-induced hyperglycemia. Endocr Pract 2016;22(2):180–9.
36. Afrezza [package insert]. Bridgewater, NJ: Sanofi; 2016.

37. Hood RD, Arakaki RA, Wysham C, et al. Two treatment approaches for human regular U-500 insulin in patients with type 2 diabetes not achieving adequate glycemic control on high-dose U-100 insulin therapy with or without oral agents: a randomized titration-to target clinical trial. Endocr Rev 2015;21(7):782–93.
38. American Diabetes Association. Glycemic targets. Sec. 5. In standards of medical care in diabetes—2016. Diabetes Care 2016;39(Suppl 1):S39–46.
39. King AB, Armstrong DU. A prospective evaluation of insulin dosing recommendations in patients with type 1 diabetes at near normal glucose control: bolus dosing. J Diabetes Sci Technol 2007;1(1):42–6.
40. Davidson PC, Hebblewhite HR, Steed RD, et al. Analysis of guidelines for basal-bolus insulin dosing: basal insulin, correction factor and carbohydrate-to-insulin ratio. Endocr Pract 2008;14(9):1095–101.

Special Considerations in Choosing Diabetes Therapy

Melissa Murfin, PA-C, PharmD, BCACP

KEYWORDS

- Diabetes treatment • Polypharmacy • Renal dosing • Special populations
- Weight neutral

KEY POINTS

- Treating diabetes across requires a different approach in pediatric and elderly patients.
- Patients with type 2 diabetes and renal insufficiency may require dose adjustment or discontinuation of medications as their renal function declines.
- Choosing medications to minimize weight gain is important for patients with type 2 diabetes who may already be struggling with weight issues.
- The risk of hypoglycemia can be minimized by careful medication choices.
- Polypharmacy can be decreased through the use of medication review tools that help to optimize treatment for patients.

INTRODUCTION

Choosing appropriate treatment for patients with diabetes can be difficult owing to the many types of insulins and several classes of noninsulin therapies available. Add into the mix a patient with a special circumstance that might affect their response to the medication, lead to a drug or disease interaction, or be an option that is too costly, and an already difficult task becomes nearly impossible. Fortunately, the variety of treatment options available means a provider can typically find a medication that suits patients' individual issues.

The American Diabetes Association (ADA) and the European Association for the Study of Diabetes listed particular areas of concern for optimizing pharmacotherapy in a 2012 position statement that recommended an individualized approach to diabetes management based on certain patient characteristics.[1] These special considerations include:

- Patient age and weight,
- Sex, racial, ethnic, genetic, and differences,

Disclosures: None.
Department of Physician Assistant Studies, Elon University, 2087 Campus Box, Elon, NC 27244, USA
E-mail address: mmurfin@elon.edu

Physician Assist Clin 2 (2017) 39–52
http://dx.doi.org/10.1016/j.cpha.2016.09.001
2405-7991/17/© 2016 Elsevier Inc. All rights reserved.

- Comorbidities such as coronary artery disease, heart failure, chronic kidney disease (CKD), and liver dysfunction,
- Risk for hypoglycemia, and
- Cost of treatment.

Another important consideration is polypharmacy. Patients taking multiple medications are at greater risk of issues owing to adverse effects, drug interactions, and difficulty with adherence to their regimens. Type 2 diabetes is 1 condition where polypharmacy very often comes into play because patients may be taking multiple medications to meet hyperglycemic goals, not to mention the drugs they may be using to treat common comorbidities such as hypertension, hyperlipidemia, heart failure, and so on.

Consideration of each of these specific issues when prescribing for patients reinforces the patient-centered approach now recognized by the ADA and the European Association for the Study of Diabetes. Ideally, this will lead to better outcomes for patients in the long term.

CHOOSING THERAPY IN THE ELDERLY

The 2012 position statement from the ADA and the European Association for the Study of Diabetes offered providers a paradigm shift in recommendations regarding treatment of patients with diabetes.[1] Glycemic goals are now more personalized depending on patient characteristics. Life expectancy is a specific circumstance where recommendations for treatment goals changed dramatically. More stringent management is suggested in patients with a longer life expectancy, such as a pediatric patient, and less strict for those with a shorter life expectancy such as a frail, geriatric patient.[1] This recommendation was maintained in the 2015 update as well.[2] However, it can be difficult to predict life expectancy in elderly patients owing to the variety of ways in which diabetes presents. Many factors are at play, including duration of diabetes and complications, additional comorbidities, and overall functionality.[3] Aside from life expectancy, elderly patients can be more difficult to manage owing to their medical complexity. The elderly often have a greater number of comorbidities leading to more complexities in prescribing and a greater risk of polypharmacy, as well as renal insufficiency owing to normal decreases with age, and the potential for social or economic concerns, such as caregiver issues and limited financial resources.[1]

Complications of hypoglycemic episodes are more of a concern in the elderly owing to a greater risk of falls and the potential for risk in a patient with unstable cardiac status.[1] There is an association reported with cardiac events and death in patients who experience severe hypoglycemia.[4] Requirements for strict management of hemoglobin A1c are relaxed from less than 7% for most diabetes patients to less than 7.5% to 8.5% for older adults to minimize the potential for hypoglycemia.[3] The American Academy of Endocrinologists and American College of Endocrinologists in their joint 2016 guidelines also suggest individualizing A1c goals with less than or equal to 6.5% recommended for most patients, but the less stringent greater than 6.5% for patients with serious comorbidities and a greater risk for hypoglycemia.[5]

Sulfonylureas/glinides and insulin are commonly associated with hypoglycemia and should be monitored closely when used in elderly patients. Patients may need to test their blood glucose more frequently when using these agents to decrease the potential for complications owing to hypoglycemia. Older patients in long-term care are particularly vulnerable to hypoglycemia and should be monitored closely to ensure appropriate treatment.[3] Glyburide (Micronase, DiaBeta, Glynase) specifically is recommended to be avoided in elderly patients owing to its long duration of action as compared with other sulfonylureas.[6] This extended action increases the potential for hypoglycemia. Sliding scale insulin should also be avoided owing to the greater risk of hypoglycemia without significant evidence of improvement in diabetes management.[6]

Many other medications for type 2 diabetes are associated with a lower risk for hypoglycemia.[5] These include:

- Metformin (Glucophage, Glumetza, Riomet);
- Dipeptidyl peptidase-4 (DPP-4) inhibitors such as alogliptin (Nesina), linagliptin (Tradjenta), saxagliptin (Onglyza), and sitagliptin (Januvia);
- Glucagonlike peptide-1 (GLP-1) agonists such as albiglutide (Tanzeum), dulaglutide (Trulicity), exenatide (Byetta, Bydureon), and liraglutide (Victoza);
- Sodium-glucose cotransporter 2 (SGLT2) inhibitors such as canagliflozin (Invokana), dapagliflozin (Farxiga), and empagliflozin (Jardiance);
- Alpha glucosidase inhibitors such as acarbose (Precose) and miglitol (Glyset);
- Thiazolidinediones such as pioglitazone (Actos) and rosiglitazone (Avandia);
- Bromocriptine (Cycloset);
- Pramlintide (Symlin); and
- Colesevelam (Welchol).

Although thiazolidinediones such as pioglitazone and rosiglitazone have a lesser risk of hypoglycemia, this drug class is associated with risk of fractures and worsening heart failure, both of which are concerns in the geriatric population and should be used with caution.[5]

The ADA recommendations for minimizing hypoglycemia in older adults with type 2 diabetes are as follows[3]:

- Metformin first-line in patients without renal insufficiency or 'significant' heart failure;
- GLP-1 agonists;
- DPP-4 inhibitors; and
- SGLT2 inhibitors.

However, there is some concern regarding the use of SGLT2 inhibitors in the elderly population owing to the lack of long-term data. The Food and Drug Administration has required an update of labeling to include the potential for diabetic ketoacidosis, urosepsis, and pyelonephritis owing to reports of ketoacidosis in 54 patients with type 2 diabetes as well as 19 cases of urosepsis and pyelonephritis.[7] Caution is also recommended in regard to using these medications in the elderly owing to concerns for hypotension in hypovolemic patients. Patients with low systolic blood pressure and who are also currently taking diuretics are recommended to be monitored and have hypovolemia corrected before starting an SGLT2 inhibitor.[8]

CHOOSING THERAPY IN CHILDREN

Diabetes in the pediatric population is typically type 1 and treated with various insulins; however, the number of children diagnosed with type 2 diabetes is increasing. It is estimated that one-third of new diabetes cases in American kids under 18 years of age are now type 2.[9] It can still be challenging to differentiate type 1 and type 2 diabetes in children, which increases the difficulty of making an appropriate choice of treatment. Guidelines from the American Academy of Pediatrics indicate type 2 diabetes is more likely in children who are overweight or obese with a strong family history of type 2 and some evidence of insulin resistance such as acanthosis nigricans or polycystic ovarian syndrome.[9] Additional diagnostic considerations include evidence of normal or elevated insulin or C-peptide levels at diagnosis, concomitant hypertension or hyperlipidemia, negative autoantibodies (ie, GAD65 antibodies, insulin autoantibodies, IA-2A), and insidious onset.[9]

Lifestyle modification is particularly critical for treatment in this population owing to the potential for longevity of the disease. This should include nutrition and exercise management as well as restrictions on non–school-related "screen time."[9] Family and/or caregivers should be included in this plan for better chance of success. Depression, peer pressure, and loss to follow-up often are barriers for patients in achieving lifestyle goals.[9] Discussing these issues with patients and formulating an action plan with the patient and their family may be helpful in maintaining adherence to these changes.

Recommendations for treatment include insulin at diagnosis in patients who present with ketosis, random blood glucose of greater than or equal to 250 mg/dL and/or hemoglobin A1c of greater than 9%, especially because it may be difficult to differentiate type 1 from uncontrolled type 2 at this point.[9] For other presentations consistent with type 2 diabetes criteria, metformin is the first-line treatment. Doses consistent with adult regimens are recommended: starting with 500 mg/d, increasing by 500 mg weekly or biweekly until achieving a maintenance dose of 1000 mg BID.[9] The goal for hemoglobin A1c in this population is recommended to be less than 7% with A1c levels monitored every 3 months.[9]

CHOOSING THERAPY TO MINIMIZE WEIGHT GAIN

Lifestyle modification and weight loss are important parts of diabetes treatment, particularly in patients with type 2 diabetes. Older treatments such as insulin, sulfonylureas, and thiazolidinediones are associated with weight gain, which can lead to difficulty maintaining blood glucose goals as well as problems with patient acceptance. Some oral and injectable medications are less likely to cause weight gain and may even contribute to weight loss, which may be aid in patients meeting their glycemic goals.

Metformin is considered to be weight neutral or even to offer modest benefits for weight loss in patients with type 2 diabetes. A study using Glucophage XR in patients who were unable to meet glucose goals on diet and exercise alone identified a weight loss of 2.2 lbs over 16 weeks as compared with weight loss of 1.8 lbs with placebo.[10] Metformin is currently being studied for weight loss in patients without diabetes as well. One study showed weight loss of 11 lbs over 1 year in women with midlife weight gain when accompanied by a diet that modified carbohydrates.[11] This was compared with women who were using the diet alone.

The GLP-1 agonists are incretin mimetics associated with weight loss. They include the following medications:

- Albiglutide,
- Dulaglutide,
- Exenatide, and
- Liraglutide (Saxenda).

This class of drugs works in response to ingested glucose and may contribute to weight loss owing to a feeling of early satiety in patients, which is a central effect of GLP-1. The medications also slow gastric emptying. Because of this, these drugs should be used cautiously in patients with preexisting gastroparesis.[12]

GLP-1 agonists are associated with greater potential for weight loss than metformin with studies showing approximately 3 kg weight loss after 26 weeks of use in patients with type 2 diabetes.[13] Liraglutide is also approved by the Food and Drug Administration under the brand name Saxenda for weight loss in patients without diabetes.[14] When liraglutide is used for weight loss, the dosing is higher than for type 2 diabetes. Patients taking liraglutide for weight loss will inject a dose of 3 mg/d versus a maximum dose of 1.8 mg/d for liraglutide.[12,14]

SGLT2 inhibitors are the newest class of medications available in the diabetes treatment armament. This class includes the following drugs:

- Canagliflozin,
- Dapagliflozin, and
- Empagliflozin.

Patients taking these medications may see some weight loss of approximately 2 kg over 6 to 12 months.[2]

There are additional medications for diabetes that may not contribute to weight loss; however, the drugs are considered to be weight neutral in that they are unlikely to cause weight gain. DPP-4 inhibitors include the medications:

- Alogliptin,
- Linagliptin,
- Saxagliptin, and
- Sitagliptin.

The DPP-4 inhibitors are considered to be weight neutral and are fairly well-tolerated. Alpha-glucosidase inhibitors like acarbose are also weight neutral; however, the significant gastrointestinal side effects that accompany this drug also make patient acceptance of treatment very difficult. Other medications for diabetes that are weight neutral include colsevelam and bromocriptine.[5]

CHOOSING THERAPY FOR PATIENTS WITH RENAL DISEASE

Kidney disease is a known complication of diabetes, occurring in patients with type 1 and type 2 diabetes. Up to 40% of patients with diabetes experience kidney damage as a result of their disease.[4,15] CKD is defined by stages related to kidney damage and estimated glomerular filtration rate (eGFR). The GFR is calculated from the patient's serum creatinine level and other factors. Many laboratories supply estimated eGFR calculations when a patient's serum creatinine is drawn (**Table 1**).

Medications that are eliminated renally require special attention for patients with kidney disease. Many can be managed with dose adjustments; however, some are

Table 1
Chronic kidney disease stages

Stage	eGFR (mL/min/1.73 m^2)	Definition
1	≥90	Kidney damage with normal or increased eGFR
2	60–89	Kidney damage with mildly decreased eGFR
3 A,B	30–59	Moderately decreased eGFR
4	15–29	Severely decreased eGFR
5	<15	Kidney failure or dialysis

Abbreviation: eGFR, estimated glomerular filtration rate.

Data from National Kidney Foundation. Inker LA, Astor BC, Fox CH, et al. KDOQI US Commentary on the 2012 KDIGO Clinical Practice Guideline for the Evaluation and Management of CKD. Am J Kidney Disease 2014;63(5):716. Accessed September 27, 2016. http://www.ajkd.org/article/S0272-6386(14)00491-0/fulltext#sec4.2.

contraindicated depending on the patient's current eGFR. Generally, insulin is relatively safe in patients with diabetes and CKD, although patients may require additional monitoring, particularly in CKD stages 4 and 5, because insulin may be processed and eliminated more slowly from the body, leading to an increased risk of hypoglycemia.[1]

For patients with type 2 diabetes, the most commonly used first-line oral and injectable medications require some attention with regard to the patient's renal status. Clinicians should start considering dosing or medication changes once the patient's eGFR is less than or equal to 60 mL/min. Historically, the metformin package insert included a contraindication in men with serum creatinine of greater than or equal to 1.5 mg/dL and women with serum creatinine of greater than or equal to 1.4 mg/dL owing to the risk of lactic acidosis.[16] There was significant concern among prescribers that this limited the use of metformin in patients who could benefit from it.[1] However, in April, 2016, the Food and Drug Administration completed a study review and relaxed this warning owing to data showing the risk of danger in patients with mild to moderate renal insufficiency is low.[17] The metformin label now includes the following recommendations[17]:

- Monitor metformin based on eGFR rather than serum creatinine.
- Obtain baseline and at least annual eGFR measurements in patients taking metformin.
- Avoid or discontinue metformin in patients whose eGFR is less than 30 mL/min.
- Do not start metformin in patients whose eGFR is less than or equal to 45 mL/min. In patients on metformin, assess risks of continuing therapy if the eGFR decreases to less than 45 mL/min.
- Hold metformin for patients with an eGFR of less than 60 mL/min before procedures involving iodinated contrast materials. Measure the eGFR 48 hours later and restart metformin if renal function is stable.

The DPP-4 inhibitors can be used in patients with CKD, although most require decreased doses as the patient's eGFR decreases.[16] Linagliptin may be a good choice in patients with CKD, because it is primarily eliminated outside the renal system. No dosing change is required for patients with renal insufficiency.[18] Sitagliptin dosing is reduced from 100 to 50 mg/d for patients with an eGFR of 30 to 50 mL/min and to 25 mg/d for patients with an eGFR of less than 30 mL/min.[16] Saxagliptin has a similar dose reduction strategy for patients with CKD, reducing the respective doses by one-half once the eGFR is less than 50 mL/min.[16] Alogliptin also requires dose reduction by half with an eGFR of 30 to less than 60 mL/min and further reduction to a quarter dose for patients with an eGFR of less than 30 mL/min.[19]

The SGLT 2 inhibitors work primarily by blocking glucose reabsorption in the kidneys, allowing for an increase in renal excretion of glucose. As a result, in patients with renal impairment, some efficacy is lost. The drugs themselves also have been shown to increase serum creatinine, although this is a transient effect. Canagliflozin, dapagliflozin, and empagliflozin are should not be used in patients with an eGFR of less than 45 mL/min with a more strict limit for dapagliflozin to avoid use with an eGFR of less than 60 mL/min.[20,21]

The GLP-1 agonists vary in recommendations for use in patients with severe CKD. Exenatide should be avoided once patients the eGFR is less than 30 mL/min.[16] Albiglutide, dulaglutide, and liraglutide have no restrictions or dose adjustments required for patients with renal impairment.[22,23]

Sulfonylureas can be used in patients with CKD; however, only glimepiride and glipizide are recommended. Glyburide and the first-generation sulfonylureas such as chlorpropamide are contraindicated owing to the possibility of increased hypoglycemia as the medication builds up in the patient's system owing to decreased elimination.[16] Thiazolidinediones are eliminated hepatically and are only a concern in CKD owing to the possibility of fluid retention.

Less common medications for type 2 diabetes can be used in patients with mild renal impairment. The alpha glucosidase inhibitor acarbose is recommended to be avoided in patients with a serum creatinine of greater than 2 mg/dL owing to lack of safety data available.[24] Colesevelam seems to have no effect on renal function, although it was not studies directly in patients with an eGFR of less than 30 mL/min.[25] Pramlintide, the amylin analog, is one of few medications labeled for use in both types 1 and 2 diabetes treatment. No dose adjustments are required when using pramlintide in patients with diabetes and renal insufficiency. The Kidney Disease Outcomes Quality Initiative guidelines recommend avoiding pramlintide in patients with stage 4 or 5 CKD.[16]

CHOOSING THERAPY BASED ON COST

Treatment of diabetes can be very expensive, because patients have to account for their medication costs along with the cost of supplies for injections and glucose monitoring. Older insulins like regular and NPH are less expensive than the newer rapid-acting and basal insulins, but are being replaced by these insulin analogs owing to their more predictable and desirable insulin action profile. For patients with type 2 diabetes, the used of multiple medications to achieve glycemic goals may place a financial burden on patients, particularly with the use of newer medications like the GLP-1 agonists, DPP-4 inhibitors, and SGLT2 inhibitors, which currently have no available generics.

For patients with type 2 diabetes, retail pharmacies like Walmart typically have metformin, glipizide, glimepiride, and glyburide on their list of medications that cost $4 for a 30-day supply. Prescribers who authorize a 90-day supply will save patients an additional $2 over the 30-day costs. Metformin is free in some supermarkets like Publix, which is located throughout the southeastern United States.[26] Becoming familiar with local retail pharmacy plans can be greatly beneficial.

DPP-4 inhibitors and SGLT2 inhibitors cost approximately $350 to $400 for a monthly supply for patients with no insurance.[27] Sitagliptin was the first DPP-4 and will likely be the first to go off-patent, allowing generic manufacturers to market the drug. However, the patents for sitagliptin expire in 2022, so it is unlikely there will be a generic available for some time.[28] The injectable GLP-1 agonists range in cost from $350 to $500 for a monthly supply (**Fig. 1**).

Older insulins such as NPH and regular are significantly less expensive than the newer insulin analogs like glargine (Lantus, Toujeo), glulisine (Apidra), and so on. New formulations are available in varying concentrations. Most insulins are available as the standard U-100 formulation with 100 U/mL, but newer insulins like degludec (Tresiba) and lispro (Humalog) are also available in a U-200 concentration; glargine is available as U-300. Insulin R is also available in a U-500 formulation for severely insulin-resistant patients. Pen formulations are preferred by patients for ease of use; however, insulin pens often cost more per unit than vials (**Fig. 2**).

Discount cards are available through websites such as Drugs.com and GoodRx. com. Many manufacturers also offer coupons on their websites for a free 30-day supply or to assist patients with private insurance with coverage of their copay up to 1 year. For patients without insurance, many of the major pharmaceutical manufacturers offer a patient assistance program where patients who meet low-income guidelines may receive their prescriptions free from the company. The Partnership for Prescription Assistance (https://www.pparx.org/) offers a website to help patients and prescribers identify the drug companies and any assistance programs available

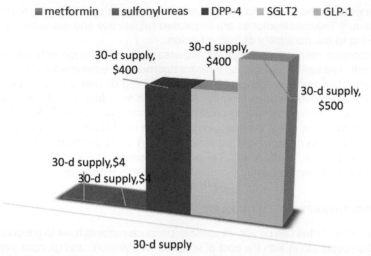

Fig. 1. Approximate 30-day drug costs for type 2 diabetes medications. DPP-4, dipeptidyl peptidase-4; GLP-1, glucagonlike peptide; SGLT2, sodium-glucose linked transporter-2. (*Data from* UpToDate. Available at: http://www.uptodate.com/home. Accessed February 18, 2016.)

for specific medications. Many of the programs require submission of tax information and authorization from the prescriber because the prescription is filled directly by the drug company or their pharmacy agent. For example, the program from Merck requires the patient's demographic information, a 90-day subscription with 3 refills, and the prescriber's signature.

CHOOSING THERAPY IN PATIENTS AT RISK FOR COMPLICATIONS OWING TO POLYPHARMACY

The term "polypharmacy" has many definitions, including patients taking 6 or more prescription medications or patients who have been prescribed inappropriate medications.[29] Patients with type 2 diabetes are estimated to take an average of 6 or more medications daily in the United States and the UK.[30] Based on current guidelines, an obese patient greater than 50 years of age presenting on initial diagnosis with an

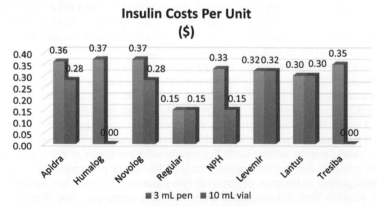

Fig. 2. Costs per insulin unit 3-mL pens and 10-mL vials of U-100 insulins. (*From* UpToDate. Available at: http://www.uptodate.com/home. Accessed February 18, 2016.)

A1c of greater than 9% may be started on 2 to 3 medications for diabetes, pharmaco-therapy for weight loss, and an aspirin for primary prevention of atherosclerotic cardio-vascular disease with the potential for additional treatment of hypertension and hyperlipidemia.[2,5] Geriatric patients are also at greater risk of complications from pol-ypharmacy owing to the likelihood of multiple comorbidities present in this population.

Concerns for complications of polypharmacy in all diabetes patients include:

- Hypoglycemia,
- Adherence,
- Cost burden,
- Complexity of dosing regimens,
- Increased potential for adverse effects, and
- Increased potential for drug interactions.

One way to prevent issues that occur for diabetes patients as a result of polypharmacy is to perform a medication review. A complete medication review should be performed on at least an annual basis for all patients as well as after a hospitalization or when a pa-tient asks for medication refills.[29,31] This can be conducted by a physician assistant or could be scheduled with a pharmacist experienced in medication therapy management.

Medication review should consist of an evaluation of all of a patient's current med-ications including prescription, over-the-counter, vitamins, minerals, and herbal sup-plements. The dose, route, timing of dosing, and indication should be confirmed for each drug along with an adverse effects the patient might be experiencing. Pre-scribers should address several areas regarding patient medications including[32]:

- Necessity,
- Contraindications particularly in the elderly or renal patients,
- Duplicate medications,
- Lowest effective dosage,
- Adverse effects,
- Simplification of drug regimen,
- Drug interactions, and
- Adherence.

Because an extensive review of this nature can take 30 to 45 minutes, a separate appointment dedicated to medication review is recommended. It is helpful to ask the patient or their caregiver to bring all of their medications for the visit to insure none are missed. There is a billable *International Classification of Disease*-10 code se-ries that may be useful for medication review reimbursement. The code—Z79 long-term (current) drug therapy—has specific drugs listed in greater detail such as Z79.4 for the long-term use of insulin whereas the code Z79.899 for other long-term (current) drug therapy may be useful for nonspecific medications.[33]

The NO TEARS mnemonic may be helpful to simplify the medication review process for busy clinicians.[34] This tool is designed to streamline the medication review and insure consistency for patients and providers. Medication review with the NO TEARS model addresses *N*ecessity and indication for each medication, *o*pen-ended ques-tions to assess patient's understanding of their treatment or any problems that might be occurring, any *t*ests and monitoring needed to ensure efficacy and safety of each drug, *e*vidence review for changes in guidelines or recommendations that might change the use of the medication, any *a*dverse effects the patient might experience, *r*isk reduction, and *s*implification of dosing regimen or switching of medications. **Table 2** combines the NO TEARS model with suggested questions for addressing each topic.

Table 2 NO TEARS medication review tool		
The NO TEARS Tool		
N	Need and indication	Is the medication still necessary? Why is the patient taking the medication?
O	Open-ended questions	Any problems with the medication? How is it working for you? Any problems getting a regular supply of medication (cost, etc)? How are you taking the medication? Can you swallow the pills and open the containers?
T	Tests and monitoring	Assess disease control Order any appropriate testing
E	Evidence and guidelines	Has the evidence or guideline changed since the medication was prescribed? Is the dose still appropriate?
A	Adverse effects	Is the patient experiencing any adverse effects from the medication? Is the patient taking a medication to treat the adverse effect of another medication?
R	Risk reduction or prevention	Any risks owing to medication use, such as fall risk, drug interactions, or inappropriate medications?
S	Simplification and switches	Can dosing be simplified or medications switched for better efficacy or adherence?

From Lewis T. Using the NO Tears tool for medication review. BMJ 2004;329:434. Available at: http://www.bmj.com/content/329/7463/434. Accessed February 11, 2016.

For example, on medication review a provider may choose to simplify a patient's regimen and decrease costs by discontinuing a DPP-4 inhibitor in a patient who is also taking a GLP-1 agonist. This could be done owing to the similar mechanisms of action between the 2 drugs.

SUMMARY

Treating patients with diabetes is not a 1-size-fits-all proposition. All patients benefit from a more individualized approach to treatment. The number of medication options available along with the attention to meeting glycemic goals means polypharmacy is likely for many patients with type 2 diabetes. More medication prescriptions along with the myriad of new, brand-only options also leads to an increased cost burden for patients. More pediatric patients are being diagnosed with type 2 diabetes, which requires tighter glycemic goals and the use of medications that may not have been studied in a pediatric population. Weight gain owing to medications is also an issue for patients with type 2 diabetes who often are struggling to lose weight. Treatment may also lead to a greater risk of hypoglycemia, which increases patients' risks of falls and cardiac issues. Patients with renal disease also have an increased risk of adverse effects; several of the diabetes medications require dose adjustment or are contraindicated in patients with renal insufficiency. Finally, elderly patients are at greater risk for many of these issues, particularly polypharmacy, hypoglycemia, and renal insufficiency, which makes treatment more complex in these patients.

Clinicians must keep all of these issues in mind to optimize treatment for their patients. It is possible that any 1 patient may be elderly with renal insufficiency, trying to lose weight, and financially disadvantaged. This certainly creates a treatment

Table 3
Choosing treatment for patients with special considerations

Drug	Low Risk of Hypoglycemia	Low Cost	No Renal Adjustments	Low Likelihood of Weight Gain	Pediatric Use
Metformin	X	X		X	X
Sulfonylureas		X			
DPP-4 inhibitors	X		Linagliptin	X	
GLP-1 agonists	X		Albiglutide Dulaglutide Liraglutide	X	
SGLT2 inhibitors	X			X	
Insulin			X		X

Abbreviations: DPP-4, dipeptidyl peptidase-4; GLP-1, glucagonlike peptide; SGLT2, sodium-glucose linked transporter-2.

challenge for the prescribing clinician. A table combining these concerns is beneficial in helping choose therapy for patients with multiple issues (**Table 3**).

With this tool, it is clear that metformin can be used in many special situations, although it may not be the best choice for patients with renal insufficiency. The DPP-4 inhibitors, GLP-1 agonists, and SGLT2 inhibitors are useful for minimizing hypoglycemic episodes and weight gain, whereas the sulfonylureas may be useful when cost is a consideration for patients. Insulin remains the best choice in renal patients.

Addressing the complexity of diabetes treatment in patients with multiple special circumstances can be difficult for providers. The use of medication review may help clinicians to identify these issues before they cause poor outcomes for patients. Using a tool that aids in streamlining this process may be beneficial in preventing adverse outcomes and complications in patients with diabetes. With careful attention to prescribing and the use of medication review, providers can manage patients with special considerations achieve their goals and prevent adverse outcomes owing to drug interactions and medication side effects.

REFERENCES

1. Inzucchi SE, Bergenstal RM, Buse JB, et al. Management of hyperglycemia in type 2 diabetes: a patient-centered approach. Position statement of the American Diabetes Association (ADA) and the European Association for the Study of Diabetes (EASD). Diabetes Care 2012;35:1364–79. Available at: http://care.diabetesjournals.org/content/35/6/1364.long. Accessed January 5, 2016.
2. Inzucchi SE, Bergenstal RM, Buse JB, et al. Management of hyperglycemia in type 2 diabetes, 2015: A patient-centered approach. Update to a position statement of the American Diabetes Association and the European Association for the Study of Diabetes. Diabetes Care 2015;38:140–9. Available at: http://care.diabetesjournals.org/content/38/1/140.full.pdf+html. Accessed December 17, 2015.
3. American Diabetes Association. Older adults. Sec. 10. In standards of medical care in diabetes—2016. Diabetes Care 2016;39(Suppl. 1):S81–5. Available at: http://care.diabetesjournals.org/content/39/Supplement_1/S81.full. Accessed January 21, 2016.
4. Handelsman Y, Bloomgarden ZT, Grunberger G, et al. American Association of Clinical Endocrinologists and American College of Endocrinology – clinical practice guidelines for developing a diabetes mellitus comprehensive care

plan – 2015. Endocr Pract 2015;21:1–87. Available at: https://www.aace.com/files/dm-guidelines-ccp.pdf. Accessed January 6, 2016.

5. Garber AJ, Abrahamson MJ, Barzilay JI, et al. Consensus statement by the American Association of Clinical Endocrinologists and American College of Endocrinology on the comprehensive type 2 diabetes management algorithm—2016 executive summary. Endocr Pract 2016;22(1):84–113. Available at: https://www.aace.com/sites/all/files/diabetes-algorithm-executive-summary.pdf. Accessed January 6, 2016.

6. American Geriatrics Society. 2015 beers criteria update expert panel. American Geriatrics Society 2015 updated Beers Criteria for potentially inappropriate medication use in older adults. J Am Geriatr Soc 2015;63:2227–46. Available at: http://onlinelibrary.wiley.com/doi/10.1111/jgs.13702/abstract. Accessed January 21, 2016.

7. FDA Drug Safety Communication. FDA revises labels of SGLT2 inhibitors for diabetes to include warnings about too much acid in the blood and serious urinary tract infections. Silver Spring, MD: U.S. Food and Drug Administration; 2015. Available at: http://www.fda.gov/Drugs/DrugSafety/ucm475463.htm. Accessed January 26, 2016.

8. Jardiance [package insert]. Ridgefield CT: Boehringer Ingelheim Pharmaceuticals, Inc; 2015. Available at: http://docs.boehringer-ingelheim.com/Prescribing%20Information/PIs/Jardiance/jardiance.pdf. Accessed January 26, 2016.

9. Copeland KC, Silverstein J, Moore KR, et al. Management of newly diagnosed type 2 diabetes mellitus (T2DM) in children and adolescents. Pediatrics 2013;131:364. Available at: http://pediatrics.aappublications.org/content/pediatrics/131/2/364.full.pdf. Accessed January 22, 2016.

10. Glucophage and Glucophage XR [package insert]. Princeton, NJ: Bristol-Myers Squibb; 2015. Available at: http://packageinserts.bms.com/pi/pi_glucophage.pdf. Accessed January 26, 2016.

11. Mogul H, Freeman R, Nguyen K. Metformin sustained weight loss and reduced android fat tissue at 12 months in EMPOWIR (Enhance the Metabolic Profile of Women with Insulin Resistance): a double-blind, placebo-controlled, randomized trial of normoglycemic women with midlife weight gain. Endocr Pract 2016;22(5):575–86. Available at: http://journals.aace.com/doi/10.4158/EP151087.OR?url_ver=Z39.88-2003&rfr_id=ori:rid:crossref.org&rfr_dat=cr_pub%3dpubmed. Accessed January 26, 2016.

12. Victoza [package insert]. Bagsvaerd, Denmark: Novo Nordisk; 2015. Available at: http://www.novo-pi.com/victoza.pdf. Accessed January 26, 2016.

13. McDougall C, McKay GA, Fisher M. Drugs for diabetes: part 6 GLP-1 receptor agonists. Br J Cardiol 2011;18:167–9. Available at: http://bjcardio.co.uk/2011/08/drugs-for-diabetes-part-6-glp-1-receptor-agonists/. Accessed January 26, 2016.

14. Saxenda [package insert]. Bagsvaerd, Denmark: Novo Nordisk; 2015. Available at: http://www.novo-pi.com/saxenda.pdf. Accessed January 26, 2016.

15. American Diabetes Association. Microvascular Complications and Foot Care. Sec. 9. In Standards of Medical Care in Diabetes—2016. Diabetes Care 2016;39(Suppl. 1):S72–80. Available at: http://care.diabetesjournals.org/content/39/Supplement_1/S72.full.pdf+html. Accessed February 1, 2016.

16. National Kidney Foundation. KDOQI Clinical practice guideline for diabetes and CKD: 2012 update. Am J Kidney Dis 2012;60(5):850–86. Available at: http://www.ajkd.org/article/S0272-6386(12)00957-2/pdf. Accessed February 1, 2016.

17. Metformin-containing drugs: drug safety communication—revised warnings for certain patients with reduced kidney function. Silver Spring, MD: U.S. Food and Drug Administration; 2016. Available at: http://www.fda.gov/safety/med watch/safetyinformation/safetyalertsforhumanmedicalproducts/ucm494829.htm. Accessed April 10, 2016.

18. Tradjenta prescribing information. Ridgefield (CT): Boehringer Ingelheim pharmaceuticals, Inc; 2015. Available at: http://docs.boehringer-ingelheim.com/Prescribing%20Information/PIs/Tradjenta/Tradjenta.pdf. Accessed February 1, 2016.

19. Nesina prescribing information. Deerfield (IL): Takeda Pharmaceuticals America, Inc; 2015. Available at: http://general.takedapharm.com/content/file.aspx?applicationcode=66b0b942-e82b-46ad-886a-f4aa59f5f33c&filetypecode=Nes inaPi&cacheRandomizer=6261e9e8-e7be-431a-bbee-7f23c667bcb8. Accessed March 17, 2016.

20. Jardiance prescribing information. Ridgefield (CT): Boehringer Ingelheim Pharmaceuticals, Inc; 2015. Available at: http://docs.boehringer-ingelheim.com/Prescribing%20Information/PIs/Jardiance/jardiance.pdf. Accessed February 2, 2016.

21. Farxiga prescribing information. Wilmington (DE): AstraZeneca Pharmaceuticals LP; 2015. Available at: http://www.azpicentral.com/farxiga/pi_farxiga.pdf. Accessed March 17, 2016.

22. Tanzeum prescribing information. Wilmington (DE): GlaxoSmithKline, LLC; 2015. Available at: https://www.gsksource.com/pharma/content/dam/GlaxoSmithKline/US/en/Prescribing_Information/Tanzeum/pdf/TANZEUM-PI-MG-IFU-COMBINED. PDF. Accessed February 18, 2016.

23. Trulicity prescribing information. Indianapolis (IN): Eli Lilly and Company; 2015. Available at: http://uspl.lilly.com/trulicity/trulicity.html#pi. Accessed February 18, 2016.

24. Acarbose drug label information. Parsippany (NJ): Arrow Pharma, Inc; Actavis Pharma, Inc; 2014. Available at: http://dailymed.nlm.nih.gov/dailymed/drugInfo. cfm?setid=6c2db888-775c-4baf-a1b4-1cfa63b83357. Accessed February 2, 2016.

25. Colesevelam drug label information. Parsippany (NJ): Daiichi Sankyo, Inc; 2014. Available at: http://dailymed.nlm.nih.gov/dailymed/drugInfo.cfm?setid=4a06d 3b2-7229-4398-baba-5d0a72f63821. Accessed February 2, 2016.

26. Publix pharmacy free medication program. Available at: http://www.publix.com/pharmacy-wellness/pharmacy/pharmacy-services/free-medication-program. Accessed February 18, 2016.

27. Lavernia F, Adkins SE, Shubrook JH. Use of oral combination therapy for type 2 diabetes in primary care: meeting individualized patient goals. Postgrad Med 2015;127(8):808–17. Available at: http://www.tandfonline.com/doi/full/10.1080/00325481.2015.1085293. Accessed February 9, 2016.

28. Generic januvia availability. Drugs.com. Available at: http://www.drugs.com/availability/generic-januvia.html. Accessed February 9, 2016.

29. Bushardt RL, Massey EB, Simpson KN, et al. Polypharmacy: misleading, but manageable. Clin Interv Aging 2008;3(2):383–9. Available at: http://www.ncbi.nlm.nih.gov/pmc/articles/PMC2546482/. Accessed February 11, 2016.

30. Black JA, Simmons RK, Boothby CE, et al. Medication burden in the first 5 years following diagnosis of type 2 diabetes: findings form the ADDITION-UK trial cohort. BMJ Open Diabetes Res Care 2015;3:e000075. Available at: http://drc. bmj.com/content/3/1/e000075.full.pdf+htm. Accessed February 11, 2016.

31. Tarn DM, Paterniti DA, Kravitz RL, et al. How do physicians conduct medication reviews? J Gen Intern Med 2008;24(12):1296–302.
32. Bushardt RL, Jones KW. Nine key questions to address polypharmacy in the elderly. JAAPA 2005;18(5):32–7. Available at: http://journals.lww.com/jaapa/Abstract/2005/05000/Nine_key_questions_to_address_polypharmacy_in_the.5.aspx?sessionEnd=true. Accessed February 11, 2016.
33. ICD10Data.com. Available at: http://www.icd10data.com/. Accessed February 11, 2016.
34. Lewis T. Using the NO TEARS tool for medication review. BMJ 2004;329:434. Available at: http://www.bmj.com/content/329/7463/434. Accessed February 11, 2016.

The Never Ending Debate
T3...Yes or No?

Sonia L. Bahroo, PA-C

KEYWORDS

- Thyroid • Hypothyroidism • Levothyroxine • Triiodothyronine • Liothyronine
- Thyroid-stimulating hormone

KEY POINTS

- There are 4 options for the treatment of hypothyroidism: levothyroxine monotherapy, liothyronine monotherapy, combination treatment with levothyroxine and liothyronine, and desiccated thyroid extracts.
- Levothyroxine is the current standard of care in hypothyroidism treatment, whereas liothyronine is a source of contention and debate.
- Unless dosed multiple times daily, liothyronine monotherapy results in unstable serum triiodothyronine (T3) levels. Slow release formulations produce more even T3 levels, but there are no formal pharmacokinetic studies.
- Research shows liothyronine can be used successfully in certain subgroups of patients.
- The American Thyroid Association Task Force on Thyroid Hormone Replacement advises against immediate release liothyronine for routine use, but supports continued research of extended release liothyronine.

INTRODUCTION

Hypothyroidism is one of the most common disorders treated in endocrinology practice. It has a prevalence of 3.8% to 4.6%, being more common in females than males. In the Western hemisphere, the most common cause of hypothyroidism is autoimmune thyroiditis, but in many other countries one of the major causes is still iodine deficiency. In addition, hypothyroidism is caused by certain drugs such as amiodarone and lithium, total thyroidectomy, and radioactive iodine therapy. It can also be congenital.[1]

Before 1891, a diagnosis of hypothyroidism was frequently fatal because it had no cure. In that year British physician George Murray subcutaneously injected sheep thyroid extract into a patient with myxedema. This was the first major milestone in the treatment of hypothyroidism. His continued work and observations eventually led to

The author has nothing to disclose.
Division of Endocrinology, Department of Medicine, The George Washington University Medical Faculty Associates, Inc, 2150 Pennsylvania Avenue Northwest, Washington, DC 20037, USA
E-mail address: sbahroo@mfa.gwu.edu

Physician Assist Clin 2 (2017) 53–60
http://dx.doi.org/10.1016/j.cpha.2016.08.006
2405-7991/17/© 2016 Elsevier Inc. All rights reserved.

the development of a desiccated thyroid extract preparation that became standard treatment for hypothyroidism and conditions requiring pituitary suppression of thyroid-stimulating hormone (TSH).[1,2]

The structure of thyroxine was identified in 1926 and it became available for commercial use in the 1930s.[1] By the 1950s, it became widely available, but did not replace the mainstay treatment of thyroid extract until the 1970s.[2] Similarly, triiodothyronine (T3) was first discovered in 1952 by Gross and Pitts-River[1]; synthetic liothyronine was used clinically by 1956.[2] See **Fig. 1** for a timeline of major breakthroughs in hypothyroidism.

Controversy exists over the use of liothyronine. We already have levothyroxine as the cornerstone of hypothyroidism treatment, so is there a need for liothyronine? One logical argument for its use is this: if one has a deficiency in thyroid hormones, why not directly replace both of them? On the other hand, the peripheral conversion of tetraiodothyronine (T4) to liothyronine T3 already occurs naturally in the body. Why interfere with that reaction by adding synthetic liothyronine? The present article seeks to address this ongoing debate.

CURRENT OPTIONS FOR TREATMENT
Levothyroxine

The thyroid gland produces both T4 and T3, but T4 in much greater quantity.[3] In fact, approximately 80% of circulating T3 is produced by peripheral monodeiodination of T4,[4] whereas only 20% is directly secreted by the thyroid gland.[5] As of 1970 it was unknown whether T4 acts on its own or only after conversion to T3.[3] It is now widely accepted that T4 acts as a prohormone of T3[2] and that T3 is more metabolically active than T4.[3]

The conversion of T4 to T3 predominantly occurs by way of the enzyme deiodinase 2.[5] Because T4 converts to T3 in vivo, taking levothyroxine alone could be sufficient to lower the TSH, normalize T4 levels, and thereby alleviate the symptoms of hypothyroidism. Therefore, there may not be a need for separate T3 supplementation.

Levothyroxine has a long half-life of 7 days, which allows for convenient, once-daily dosing. The most common method for initiating levothyroxine therapy is to start at a low dose and titrate upward over weeks to several months. This method works well and is safe to use in cases of subclinical, mild, and overt hypothyroidism. The downside for patients is that this requires multiple laboratory visits for blood draws; for providers, it demands regular follow-up with patients to report laboratory results and adjust dosage. Interestingly, a randomized trial by Roos and colleagues[6] in 2005 showed that initial dosing based on body weight can be safe, efficient, and use less resources compared with the typical approach. For full replacement therapy in overt hypothyroidism, dosing based on body weight is done at 1.6 μg/kg per day in healthy, nonpregnant patients. For the elderly and those patients with ischemic heart disease, however, the traditional approach would be safer.[1]

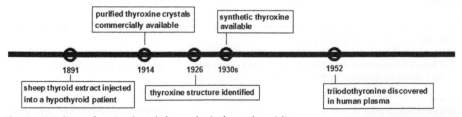

Fig. 1. Timeline of major breakthroughs in hypothyroidism.

Steady-state hormone levels are usually achieved about 6 weeks after the initiation of levothyroxine therapy or after any adjustments in dosage.[5] Therefore, the TSH level must be monitored at these intervals and then typically on an annual basis once a stable dose is achieved. The goal of therapy is to maintain TSH in the lower one-half of the normal reference range, up to about 2.5 mU/L.[1] If there is difficulty in achieving the target TSH, providers should verify adherence not only with taking the medication but taking it correctly.[7] It is best absorbed when taken on an empty stomach at least one hour before food intake and must be separated from calcium, iron, and any medications or supplements containing these ingredients by at least 4 hours. It is noteworthy to point out that even in an optimal fasting state levothyroxine absorption is only approximately 70% to 80%. One study found absorption decreased to about 64% with the presence of food.[5] Absorption of levothyroxine is also decreased in the presence of certain gastrointestinal conditions such as malabsorption syndromes, celiac disease, and gastritis.[4,5]

Levothyroxine is typically taken first thing in the morning, but if patients find it difficult to be adherent with this they can take it at nighttime as long as they wait 3 or more hours after food intake.[5,7] Another possibility for patients who have difficulty adhering to a daily administration schedule is to take a once weekly oral dose of levothyroxine that is 7 times the usual daily dose. This may be helpful in elderly patients who are dependent on caregivers or visiting nurses. Taking it once weekly has been shown to result in T4 peaks for about 24 hours, with T3 levels staying within the reference range.[1]

It is important to explain to patients that it may take several months for symptoms to improve or resolve after thyroid laboratory values normalize.[7] Patients should also be advised to remain on the same brand or generic preparation of levothyroxine for the duration of therapy, which is usually lifelong. This is a key factor in maintaining normal and consistent target blood levels of thyroid hormones. In an ideal world, all formulations of levothyroxine would be bioequivalent, but unfortunately this is not the case in reality. If a change in brand or generic formulation occurs, the TSH level should be tested 6 weeks later.[5] Although that is not the primary focus of this article, there is extensive discussion about this topic and it is, therefore, worth mentioning.

In their 2014 Guidelines for the Treatment of Hypothyroidism, the American Thyroid Association Task Force on Thyroid Hormone Replacement (ATA Task Force) advocates the use of levothyroxine as their choice preparation. It is inexpensive, effective, easy to take, and well absorbed. Furthermore, it has a long half-life, a good side effect profile, and excellent long-term benefits data.[5]

Liothyronine

T3 levels are known to be low in extremes of age, starvation, hepatic and renal dysfunction, perisurgical state, and chronic disease.[4] Some of these conditions would be categorized as euthyroid sick syndrome so would not warrant thyroid hormone replacement therapy. There is a lack of data on the physiologic effects when T3 is in the low-normal or below reference range.[5]

Current clinical practice dictates normalization of TSH as the goal of therapy for hypothyroidism. Serum total and free T3 levels are not tested routinely. Hormone replacement using levothyroxine depends on the successful conversion of T4 to T3. A defect in this reaction would cause insufficient production of T3. Taking liothyronine directly bypasses this step. It delivers drug directly to its target tissues and organs; however, it inhibits extrathyroidal deiodination reactions because T4 would not be present to serve as the substrate.[5]

Unlike levothyroxine sodium, which is heavily protein bound, liothyronine sodium is not, so it is more bioavailable compared with levothyroxine. It does not have to be taken in a fasting state. This results in a rapid onset of action (occurring within a few hours of ingestion). Maximal pharmacologic response occurs in 2 to 3 days, consequently producing quick clinical response. Liothyronine tablets are available in 3 strengths: 5, 25, and 50 μg. Its half-life is approximately 1 to 2.5 days.[5,8] It is also available as an intravenous solution (Triostat) for the treatment of myxedema coma or pre-coma in adults.[9]

The results of a double-blind randomized cross-over study indicated that liothyronine was as equally effective as levothyroxine in suppressing serum TSH level when it was administered 3 times a day at an levothyroxine (LT4):liothyronine (LT3) ratio of 1:3. This study was complicated; on average, it took 6 months and several dose adjustments to achieve the target TSH. Based on the results of this study, the ATA Task Force does not support liothyronine monotherapy in its current immediate release formulation because it cannot provide steady T3 levels. The ATA Task Force does state that liothyronine monotherapy may seem advantageous in the setting of obesity and dyslipidemia. However, there is presently not enough evidence to determine whether it is more effective than therapy with levothyroxine owing to concerns over adherence and toxicity.[5]

A disadvantage to monotherapy with liothyronine is that it results in serum T3 concentration peaks and troughs owing to its short half-life. Multiple daily dosing would have to be implemented to provide steady levels, but this would likely decrease adherence. A study by Hennemann and colleagues showed promising results with sustained release formulation of liothyronine. The details of this study are discussed in Combination Therapy with LT4 and LT3. The ATA Task Force recommends clinical trials of a longer duration using a longer acting form of liothyronine before it can support this agent for routine use. Additionally, monotherapy with liothyronine is more expensive compared with levothyroxine.[5]

Combination Therapy with LT4 and LT3

In studies of thyroidectomized rats, only combination treatment with levothyroxine and liothyronine adequately achieved euthyroid levels in all tissues; levothyroxine monotherapy was not able to do so. These findings can be extrapolated to humans[10]; however, multiple studies in humans have demonstrated that combination treatment is not advantageous clinically to monotherapy with levothyroxine.[1,10,11] This was also the outcome of a 2002 study done by Cassio and colleagues,[12] which was done on neonates with congenital hypothyroidism.

It is unknown then why a small subset of hypothyroid patients still experience symptoms of hypothyroidism despite being treated optimally with levothyroxine. A recent study shows a positive correlation between hypothyroid patients treated with levothyroxine who have a genetic variation in the deiodinase 2 (DIO2) gene and worse baseline quality-of-life scores. It seems that these patients respond better to combination therapy with liothyronine.[1,10] There is also evidence that the presence of thyroid peroxidase antibodies, even after a patient becomes euthyroid, is more associated with having residual symptoms than those without thyroid autoimmunity.[5]

In a study done by Nygaard and colleagues,[11] 49% of patients preferred combination therapy over monotherapy with levothyroxine. The patients they tested who had a high baseline psychological morbidity and autoimmune hypothyroidism seemed to do better on combination therapy with levothyroxine and liothyronine. The study authors noted a direct relationship between combination therapy and test scores for quality of life and depression.

A 2001 study by Appelhof and colleagues[10] showed patient preference for combination treatment not owing to improvement in their secondary outcome endpoints, which included neurocognitive tests and questionnaires about quality of life and subjective symptoms, but owing to satisfaction of weight loss by study medication. Weight loss by itself was not an endpoint in this study. The study had 3 treatment arms: (1) levothyroxine alone, (2) levothyroxine and liothyronine in a ratio of 10:1, and (3) levothyroxine and liothyronine in a ratio of 5:1. The greater the T3 amount that was received, the greater the weight loss and subsequent level of satisfaction. Weight gain is a common complaint of hypothyroid patients, so it would seem logical that patients who lost weight while taking study medication were satisfied with its use. One major limitation of this study is that combination therapy resulted in overreplacement in many patients. The authors did not feel their results supported the use of combination therapy as standard treatment of hypothyroidism.

These studies give more credibility to the notion that there are patient populations that can likely benefit from the addition of liothyronine. These subgroups may include those who have the genetic variation of the DIO2 gene, psychological comorbidities, and obesity. Additional research with each of these patient subgroups would certainly be beneficial.

Another special population to consider for combination treatment is patients who are athyroid after thyroidectomy, such as those with thyroid cancer. These patients no longer have the ability to produce intrathyroidal T3. More studies are needed to determine if combination treatment is a viable treatment option in this scenario because the studies thus far have been limited in quantity and number of patients.[5]

A downside of using combination therapy is that it can result in overtreatment, that is, reduction of TSH level below the normal reference range. This has been seen in multiple studies.[1,10,11] Overtreatment can lead to unwanted side effects associated with thyrotoxicosis, such as palpitations or tremors, as well as increase the risk for atrial fibrillation and osteoporosis.[10]

One possible way to combat the problem of overtreatment is by using a slow release version of liothyronine, which is available at compounding pharmacies.[10] Studies have been done to see if this is worth further pursuit. Because regular liothyronine has such a quick onset of action and short half-life, the study by Appelhof and associates[10] dosed it twice daily to minimize nonphysiologic peaks in serum T3 levels. In another study, Hennemann and colleagues[13] concluded that treatment with levothyroxine and slow release liothyronine resulted in improved laboratory values of TSH, T4, T3, and T4:T3 ratio compared with treatment with levothyroxine alone. As they predicted, it also did not result in peaks of T3 serum levels. Based on this study, Wartofsky[14] acknowledged a slow release T3 preparation could be of significant value in the market.

The ATA Task Force suggests that, if a patient on levothyroxine with normal TSH still has symptoms or if T3 level is slightly low, there are 2 options: (1) increase levothyroxine dose (which would increase T3 level) or (2) slightly reduce levothyroxine dose and add low-dose liothyronine to normalize circulating T3 without necessarily lowering TSH.[5] Adding liothyronine should be temporary; one study did not show sustained long-term benefits. Overall, the ATA Task Force does not support the use of combination treatment as routine therapy owing to conflicting data.[5]

Desiccated Thyroid Extract

Desiccated pig thyroid extract is commercially available as Armour thyroid. It is much more expensive than levothyroxine.[7] Because it is an animal extract, the tablets have a strong odor. It contains a combination of T4 and T3 in a ratio of approximately 4:1. The physiologic ratio of T4:T3 in humans is slightly greater than 13:1,[4] so pig extract contains much more T3 than what circulates in the human body.[1]

Aside from the points noted, a reason endocrinologists do not favor using desiccated thyroid extract is owing to the variability of thyroid hormone content between batches and lots. To resolve this issue, Armour thyroid has published the following on their website:

> Note that the amount of thyroid hormone in the thyroid gland may vary from animal to animal. To ensure that Armour Thyroid tablets are the same from tablet to tablet and lot to lot, the amount of T_4 and T_3 is measured in both the raw material and in the actual tablets.[15]

Despite its drawbacks, some patients may prefer desiccated thyroid extract because it is naturally derived as opposed to a synthetic compound. Like levothyroxine, desiccated thyroid extract is taken on a once daily regimen.[4] A randomized, double-blind, crossover study by Hoang and colleagues[16] demonstrated 48.6% of patients preferred treatment with desiccated thyroid extract over levothyroxine alone. They reported improvement in subjective symptoms such as sleep, concentration, happiness, and energy level while on desiccated thyroid extract.

Dosing of desiccated thyroid extract tablets is rather confusing. The tablets are dosed in grains corresponding to milligram equivalents.[4] Unfortunately, these milligram amounts do not correspond to the microgram amounts contained in levothyroxine or liothyronine tablets. For example, a 1-grain tablet is 60 to 65 mg, depending on the brand of extract. Each grain provides 38 µg levothyroxine (T4) and 9 µg liothyronine (T3).[5] This can make it challenging for providers to titrate and achieve goal TSH as well as to switch patients from desiccated thyroid extract to levothyroxine or vice versa.

The ATA Task Force favors the use of levothyroxine over thyroid extracts as routine treatment for primary hypothyroidism. The ATA Task Force is strongly against the use of desiccated thyroid extract during pregnancy owing to the grave complications that could arise from extract preparations with lower T4 concentrations than synthetic levothyroxine.[5]

SUMMARY

The standard of care for quite some time has been to treat hypothyroidism by using monotherapy with levothyroxine. There does, however, seem to be a place for therapy with liothyronine. Even though optimal euthyroid levels of TSH and free T4 are attained in most patients, there will be a subset of patients who may still complain of experiencing symptoms related to hypothyroidism. One could argue that their symptoms may be due to a nonthyroid etiology. For example, depression or anemia can often mimic certain features of hypothyroidism. In these cases, a simple test to measure serum T3 level could easily be ordered to distinguish between a nonthyroid cause versus "T3 hypothyroidism." In the author's clinical experience, liothyronine has been used successfully in patients with T3 level near or below normal range who complain of residual symptoms. It was discontinued when normal T3 levels were sustained.

A combination drug with the proper human physiologic concentrations of T4:T3 ratio could be an ideal way to treat hypothyroidism, specifically for those patients who exhibit residual symptoms of hypothyroidism after being treated adequately with levothyroxine. Others have suggested doing genetic studies to determine which patients would be good candidates for combination therapy. Additional future research initiatives can include better understanding of the clinical significance of low T3 levels and more studies using sustained release liothyronine.

Development of a transdermal thyroid hormone patch (levothyroxine or combination T4:T3 patch) is a novel concept to entertain. It would be convenient, effective, increase adherence by eliminating the need to fast, remove gastrointestinal absorption issues, and provide steady hormone levels. Other hormone drug therapies are available in patch form … why not thyroid hormones? Considering levothyroxine is one of the most prescribed drugs in the country, there may be a market for patients who may want to take it in a more convenient formulation. A liothyronine patch could be a useful alternative to an oral sustained release formulation. Better yet, a combination T4:T3 patch in the proper physiologic concentrations would give us the best of both worlds.

REFERENCES

1. Chakera AJ, Pearce SH, Vaidya B. Treatment for primary hypothyroidism: current approaches and future possibilities. Drug Des Devel Ther 2012;6:1–11.
2. Oppenheimer JH, Braverman LE, Toft A, et al. A therapeutic controversy. Thyroid hormone treatment: when and what? J Clin Endocrinol Metab 1995;80(10): 2873–83.
3. Braverman LE, Ingbar SH, Sterling K. Conversion of thyroxine to triiodothyronine in athyreotic human subjects. J Clin Invest 1970;49:855–64.
4. Package Insert of Armour Thyroid. Available at: http://www.allergan.com/assets/pdf/armourthyroid_pi. Accessed June 11, 2016.
5. Jonklaas J, Bianco AC, Bauer AJ, et al, American Thyroid Association Task Force on Thyroid Hormone Replacement. Guidelines for the treatment of hypothyroidism: prepared by the American Thyroid Association task force on thyroid hormone replacement. Thyroid 2014;24(12):1670–751.
6. Roos A, Linn-Rasker SP, van Domburg RT, et al. The starting dose of levothyroxine in primary hypothyroidism treatment: a prospective, randomized, double-blind trial. Arch Intern Med 2005;165(15):1714–20.
7. Vaidya B, Pearce SH. Clinical review-management of hypothyroidism in adults. BMJ 2008;337(7664):284–9.
8. Package Insert of Cytomel. Available at: http://labeling.pfizer.com/ShowLabeling.aspx?id=703. Accessed June 11, 2016.
9. Package Insert of Triostat. Available at: http://www.parsterileproducts.com/products/assets/pdf/PI/2015/PI-Triostat.pdf. Accessed June 11, 2016.
10. Appelhof BC, Fliers E, Wekking EM, et al. Combined therapy with levothyroxine and liothyronine in two ratios, compared with levothyroxine monotherapy in primary hypothyroidism: a double-blind, randomized, controlled clinical trial. J Clin Endocrinol Metab 2005;90(5):2666–74.
11. Nygaard B, Jensen EW, Kvetny J, et al. Effect of combination therapy with thyroxine (T4) and 3, 5, 3′-triiodothyronine versus T4 monotherapy in patients with hypothyroidism, a double-blind, randomised cross-over study. Eur J Endocrinol 2009;161:895–902.
12. Cassio A, Cacciari E, Cicognani A, et al. Treatment for congenital hypothyroidism: thyroxine alone or thyroxine plus triiodothyronine? Pediatrics 2003;111(5): 1055–60.
13. Hennemann G, Docter R, Visser TJ, et al. Thyroxine plus low-dose, slow-release triiodothyronine replacement in hypothyroidism: proof of principle. Thyroid 2004; 14(4):271–5.

14. Wartofsky L. Combined levotriiodothyronine and levothyroxine therapy for hypo-thyroidism: are we a step closer to the magic formula? Thyroid 2004;14(4):247–8.
15. Armour thyroid. Available at: http://www.armourthyroid.com. Accessed June 11, 2016.
16. Hoang TD, Olsen CH, Mai VQ, et al. Desiccated thyroid extract compared with levothyroxine in the treatment of hypothyroidism: a randomized, double-blind, crossover study. J Clin Endocrinol Metab 2013;98(5):1982–90.

Low Thyroid-Stimulating Hormone: What Is Next?

 CrossMark

Karen Beer, PA-C, MSPAS, RD, LD, CDE

KEYWORDS

- Hyperthyroidism • Thyroid storm • Graves disease • Thyroiditis
- Thyroid-stimulating hormone (TSH) • Free thyroxine (FT4) • Antithyroid drugs (ATDs)

KEY POINTS

- The most common causes of a low serum level of thyroid-stimulating hormone are excessive levothyroxine replacement, nonthyroidal illness, and subclinical hyperthyroidism.
- The most common cause of hyperthyroidism is Graves disease.
- Untreated thyrotoxicosis can result in weight loss, osteoporosis, atrial fibrillation, emboli, cardiovascular collapse, and death.

INTRODUCTION

The appropriate screening test for thyroid dysfunction is serum thyroid-stimulating hormone (TSH) (**Box 1; Table 1**). A TSH within the normal range excludes primary thyroid disease.[1] Causes of low TSH include increased synthesis of thyroid hormone, excessive release of preformed thyroid hormones, or an endogenous or exogenous extrathyroidal source. Excessive thyroid hormone production may be caused by Graves disease, toxic multinodular goiter (TMG), or toxic adenoma (TA). Thyroiditis, which results in release of preformed thyroid hormone, may be painless or painful.

In the United States, the prevalence of hyperthyroidism is approximately 1.3%.[2] Classic symptoms of hyperthyroidism include heat intolerance, palpitations, anxiety, fatigue, weight loss, and irregular menses in women. Clinical findings include tremor, tachycardia, stare, lid lag, and warm, moist skin.[3] When caused by overproduction, treatment with antithyroid medications, radioactive iodine (RAI) ablation, and thyroidectomy are treatment options.[4]

THYROID-STIMULATING HORMONE

The appropriate screening test for thyroid dysfunction is serum TSH. It has the highest sensitivity and specificity of any test used in the evaluation of hyperthyroidism.[5] A TSH within the normal range excludes primary thyroid disease.[1]

Disclosure: None.
Oregon Medical Group, 974 Cabriole Ct., Eugene, OR 97401, USA
E-mail address: kbeer@oregonmed.net

Physician Assist Clin 2 (2017) 61–72
http://dx.doi.org/10.1016/j.cpha.2016.08.013
2405-7991/17/© 2016 Elsevier Inc. All rights reserved.

Box 1
Causes of thyrotoxicosis based on radioactive iodine uptake

Normal or elevated uptake

Graves disease

Toxic adenoma

Toxic multinodular adenoma

Low or absent uptake

Painless thyroiditis
  Postpartum
  Amiodarone
  Lithium
  Interferon-α
  Interleukin-2

Subacute thyroiditis

Acute thyroiditis

Surreptitious intake/excessive replacement

Data from Bahn RS, Burch HB, Cooper DS, et al. Hyperthyroidism and other causes of thyrotoxicosis: management guidelines of the American Thyroid Association and American Association of Clinical Endocrinologists. Thyroid 2011;21:593–646.

Table 1
Laboratory tests for hyperthyroidism

Cause	TSH	FT4, T3	RAI Uptake/Scan	Other Helpful Tests
Graves disease	↓	↑↑	Homogenous, ↑ or N	TRAbs
SH	↓	N	Homogenous, ↑ or N if due to Graves disease; focal ↑ uptake if due to TA	TRAbs, ultrasound
TA	↓	N or ↑	Focal ↑ uptake; rest of gland may have ↓ uptake	Ultrasound
TMG	↓	N or ↑	Heterogeneous, N or ↑	Ultrasound or CT
Subacute thyroiditis	↓	↑	↓ uptake	ESR
Radiocontrast dye	↓	↑	↓↓ uptake	Urinary iodine excretion
Amiodarone	↓	↑	↓↓ uptake	Urinary iodine excretion
Surreptitious intake/ excessive replacement	↓	↑	↓ uptake	Serum Tg
Secondary (pituitary or hypothalamic disorder)	↓, ↑, or N	↓		Pituitary hormones, pituitary MRI

Data from Castro RC, Gharib H. Thyroid disorders. In: Evidence-based endocrinology. 3rd edition. Philadelphia: Lippincott William and Wilkins; 2012.

A low TSH should prompt the provider to perform a detailed medical history and physical examination. Recent illness, pregnancy, thyrotoxic symptoms, personal and family history of thyroid disease, and medication history should be questioned. Medications of interest include levothyroxine, amiodarone, lithium, interferon-α, interleukin-2, and the monoclonal antibodies used in the treatment of melanoma, ipilimumab, and nivolumab. The physical examination should include vital signs: body weight, pulse rate, blood pressure, and respiratory rate. The thyroid gland should be assessed for size, symmetry, nodularity, and tenderness. Pulmonary, cardiac, and neuromuscular function should be evaluated. One should look for peripheral edema, tremor, warm, moist skin, tachycardia, and atrial fibrillation, as well as signs specific to Graves disease, including myxedema, proptosis, eyelid retraction, and lid lag.[6]

ADDITIONAL TESTS

When the TSH is low, free thyroxine (FT4) and total triiodothyronine (T3) levels should be measured. If the TSH is low and the FT4 is elevated, thyrotoxicosis is present and Graves disease is the most common cause, followed by TMG. Normal FT4 and T3 signify subclinical hyperthyroidism (SH). T3 elevation alone is referred to as "T3 thyrotoxicosis" and may represent the earliest stage of thyroid disease or an autonomously functioning thyroid nodule.[1,6]

When the diagnosis is unclear, a radioactive iodine uptake (RAIU) is recommended, except during pregnancy or breastfeeding. Using a gamma probe, an RAIU measures how much radioactive isotope is taken up by the thyroid gland over a 24-hour period following ingestion of a technetium or RAI tracer. It demonstrates either increased or decreased uptake and differentiates various causes of thyrotoxicosis.[7,8] Normal uptake ranges from 15% to 25% at 24 hours. It is elevated in Graves disease, TA, and TMG, and decreased (0% to 2%) in thyroiditis.[4] RAIU is commonly performed together with a thyroid scan.[8]

A thyroid scan shows the distribution of radiotracer in the gland and identifies hot and cold nodules. Images are taken at 4 to 6 hours and again at 24 hours.[4,9] Homogenous distribution indicates Graves disease, whereas focal accumulation suggests TA. If there are many focal areas of uptake, the diagnosis is likely TMG.[4]

Iodinated radiocontrast agents commonly used for computed tomographic (CT) scans saturate iodine binding sites in the thyroid, rendering the uptake and scan uninterpretable. Therefore, RAIU should not be done within 8 weeks of a test using radiocontrast dye. When the duration since exposure is in question, urinary iodine assessment may be helpful.[6] Amiodarone also makes interpretation of RAIU and scan difficult due to its high iodine content. RAI is contraindicated in pregnancy and breastfeeding.

Other tests that may be helpful include TSH receptor antibodies (TRAbs), thyroid peroxidase antibodies (TPO Abs), and serum thyroglobulin (Tg). TRAbs can be found in most patients with Graves disease, but positive antibodies are not required to make the diagnosis. Measurement of TRAbs is helpful when thyroid scan and uptake are unavailable or contraindicated.[6] TPO Abs are the most sensitive (but not specific) marker of autoimmune thyroid disease. Eighty-five percent of patients with Graves disease have detectable levels. Serum Tg reflects thyroid tissue mass and physical damage or inflammation of the gland. An elevated level is a nonspecific indicator of thyroid dysfunction.

THYROTOXICOSIS

Elevated serum FT4 and T3 indicate overt thyrotoxicosis.[6] Causes of thyrotoxicosis include Graves disease, SH, TMG, TA, thyroiditis, and factitious thyroid hormone ingestion. Signs and symptoms of overt and SH are similar and may not correlate with the degree of T3 and FT4 abnormality.[10] In addition, goiter size, obstructive symptoms, and Graves ophthalmopathy may not match the severity of other symptoms. Symptoms are more pronounced in young patients and those with large goiters and are less pronounced in the elderly.[6]

Thyrotoxicosis is associated with negative cardiovascular, musculoskeletal, dermatologic, and gastrointestinal effects. Excessive thyroid hormone causes increased thermogenesis and metabolic rate and reduces serum cholesterol levels and systemic vascular resistance. Untreated thyrotoxicosis can result in weight loss, osteoporosis, atrial fibrillation, emboli, cardiovascular collapse, and death.[6] Untreated thyrotoxicosis during pregnancy increases risk of fetal and maternal complications.[3]

GRAVES DISEASE

Graves disease is responsible for 60% to 80% of hyperthyroidism. It is up to 10 times more common in women than in men and most commonly occurs between ages 40 and 60 years.[7] TRAbs stimulate TSH receptors to increase production of thyroid hormone. Increased production of thyroid hormone causes new nodules to form, existing nodules to enlarge, and nodules to become autonomous.[6] Symmetric enlargement of the thyroid (present in 90%), recent onset of ophthalmopathy (present in 30% to 50%), and moderate to severe hyperthyroidism strongly suggest Graves disease, and further search for a cause is unnecessary.[1,3,6,7] Graves ophthalmopathy consists of protrusion of the eyes, periorbital soft tissue swelling, and inflammatory changes of the extraocular muscles that result in diplopia and muscle imbalance.[3]

The RAIU pattern seen in Graves disease is elevated and diffuse.[6] TRAbs are often positive.[3]

Graves disease is treated with antithyroid drugs (ATDs), methimazole (MMI) or propylthiouracil (PTU), RAI ablation, or surgery.

TOXIC MULTINODULAR GOITER AND TOXIC ADENOMAS

TMG is more common in women, the elderly, and regions with iodine deficiency.[3,6,7] Patients have firm, heterogeneous goiters of any size.[7] RAIU in a patient with TMG shows areas of focal increased and decreased uptake.[3] If many nodules are autonomous, the pattern may be difficult to distinguish from Graves.[6]

Patients with TMG may be treated with either RAI ablation or thyroidectomy with the goal of rapidly and permanently eliminating hyperthyroidism. The risk of treatment failure is very low with near-total or total thyroidectomy, and euthyroidism is reached within days of surgery. The risk of treatment failure with RAI ablation, however, is 20%, and patients may wait months to feel better. Fifty percent to 60% will achieve euthyroidism by 3 months following RAI and 80% by 6 months. On the other hand, patients who undergo total thyroidectomy require lifelong thyroid replacement. Complications of thyroidectomy include risk of permanent hypoparathyroidism and recurrent laryngeal nerve injury. Preference for surgery should be considered in the following cases: signs or symptoms of compression, risk of coexisting thyroid cancer or hyperparathyroidism requiring surgery, large goiter, substernal or retrosternal extension, or a need to rapidly correct the thyrotoxic state. Preference should be given to RAI treatment when the patient is of advanced age, has significant comorbidity, there has been previous surgery or scarring of the neck, RAI ablation will be sufficient to treat, or there is limited access to a high-volume thyroid surgeon.[6]

TAs are benign tumors that secrete excess thyroid hormone autonomously.[3] Physical examination may reveal a palpable nodule.[3,7] Ophthalmopathy and other signs of

Graves disease are absent.[3] The RAIU pattern shows focal uptake in the adenoma but suppressed uptake in surrounding and contralateral tissue.[6] Patients may undergo surgical resection or RAI ablation. The failure rate for thyroid lobectomy or isthmusectomy is less than 1%, whereas for Iodine-131 (^{131}I), it is 5.5% to 18%. Euthyroid state is typically reached within days following surgery. Complications of thyroidectomy include risk of permanent hypoparathyroidism and recurrent laryngeal nerve injury.[6]

THYROIDITIS: SUBACUTE AND PAINLESS

Subacute thyroiditis results from release of preformed thyroid hormone, often due to viral infection. It is characterized by thyroid pain and an erythrocyte sedimentation rate (ESR) greater than 50.[1,3,6,11] The gland is firm or hard, and patients may have fever. TPO Abs are positive. RAIU demonstrates little or no uptake of the radioactive isotope. Most patients develop transient hypothyroidism, but eventually return to normal thyroid function.[3] The goal of treatment is symptom relief. β-Blockers are given for thyrotoxic symptoms, and nonsteroidal anti-inflammatory agents or salicylates are given for thyroid gland pain. Some patients may require steroids given as 40 mg of prednisone, tapered over 4 to 6 weeks.[12]

Painless thyroiditis commonly occurs postpartum, but may occur in association with medications, including amiodarone, lithium, interferon-α, and interleukin-2.[1,3,6] Painless lymphocytic thyroiditis occurs in up to 10% of women after giving birth.[3] It is caused by autoimmune thyroid tissue destruction and release of preformed hormone into the circulation. It results in a transient, self-limiting thyrotoxic state. RAIU is near zero. Patients often have a personal or family history autoimmune thyroid disease and positive TPO antibodies. Thyroid function returns to normal within 12 to 18 months in 80% of patients. These patients may also develop transient hypothyroidism before returning to normal.[3,6,11,12] β-Blockers may be helpful in controlling thyrotoxic symptoms.[11,12]

SUBCLINICAL HYPERTHYROIDISM

When the TSH is low, but FT4 levels are normal, SH is likely. It should be documented that it is a persistent problem by repeating laboratory tests in 3 to 6 months.[6] In the earliest phase, 2% to 5% of patients will have elevated T3 but normal FT4 (T3 toxicosis).[1] SH may be caused by Graves disease or an autonomously functioning thyroid nodule that secretes excessive thyroid hormone. The excessive production is sufficient to suppress pituitary secretion of TSH, but not so high as to result in an elevation of circulating thyroid hormone. It is more common in women and the elderly. Younger patients and those with autonomous nodules have a higher likelihood of progression to overt hyperthyroidism. Between 1% and 3% of elderly patients will progress to overt hyperthyroidism.[1,6]

Risks of SH include atrial fibrillation and bone loss. Risk of atrial fibrillation is nearly doubled in those with low but detectable TSH. Older men and postmenopausal women with SH have a 3- to 4-fold increase in hip fracture. Dementia may also be more common.[1] A meta-analysis found a 24% increase in mortality associated with SH.[13]

Patients older than 65 years should be treated when TSH is persistently less than 0.1 mU/L, or TSH is less than normal and there are cardiac risk factors or symptoms of thyrotoxicosis. Postmenopausal women at risk of osteoporosis and younger people with osteoporosis should also be treated.[6] Patients should be followed annually with TSH and FT4 to identify conversion to overt hyperthyroidism. Patients should be advised with low TSH but normal FT4 and T3 to ask for testing if they develop symptoms.[1]

NONTHYROIDAL ILLNESS

Acute severe illness alters thyroid hormone deiodination via cytokines, resulting in modifications to the TSH, FT4, and T3. Low TSH levels in hospitalized patients are 3 times more common due to nonthyroidal illness. Thyroid function testing should be avoided during illness or hospitalization unless thyroid dysfunction is thought to be the cause of illness.[1] If TSH is low, FT4 and T3 levels should be checked. If normal, they should be rechecked 6 to 8 weeks after the patient is stabilized or has recovered from current illness.

OTHER POPULATIONS

A US study found that 4% of blacks have TSH levels less than the reference range, compared with 1.4% of whites. Smokers also have lower TSH levels. Elderly patients have a wider distribution at both the top and the bottom ends of the range than younger patients.[1] Values return to normal in approximately 50% of patients within 5 years.[14]

Human chorionic gonadotrophin has a thyrotrophic action, resulting in lower TSH levels in the first trimester of pregnancy.[1,6] TSH levels are often low during the first trimester. These findings do not indicate hyperthyroidism and do not require treatment.[4] One should keep in mind that reference ranges during pregnancy are different than for the general public.[6]

Acute psychosis and high altitude can cause inhibition of conversion from T4 to T3.[6]

MEDICATIONS

Drugs that can alter thyroid hormone levels include amiodarone, lithium, interferon-α, interleukin-2, glucocorticoids, dopamine, propranolol, heparin, methamphetamine, ipilimumab, and nivolumab.

Patients who begin amiodarone therapy should first undergo thyroid evaluation with physical examination and laboratory testing, including TSH, FT4, T3, and TPO antibodies. Amiodarone is nearly 40% iodine by weight and is structurally similar to thyroid hormones. It is lipophilic and has a long half-life. Patients who take amiodarone ingest 20 to 40 times more than the typical daily dietary iodine intake. Amiodarone can cause both hypothyroidism and hyperthyroidism. It can inhibit synthesis of T3 from T4, destroy thyroid tissue directly, or potentiate thyroid autoimmunity in patients with Graves disease. In type I amiodarone–induced thyrotoxicosis (AIT), patients have underlying thyroid abnormalities, and iodine excess leads to excessive hormone synthesis. Patients with type I AIT may have multinodular or diffuse goiters and RAIU may be normal, elevated, or low (given the high iodine content of amiodarone). It is treated with 30 to 60 mg daily of MMI. Many will eventually require definitive treatment with RAI or thyroidectomy.[13,15]

In type II AIT, amiodarone causes thyroid follicle destruction, resulting in thyroiditis.[16] As many as 5% to 10% of patients treated with amiodarone will develop painless thyroiditis.[6] In type II AIT, the thyroid is small, diffuse, firm, and occasionally tender, and RAIU is low or absent. Type II AIT is treated with 40 to 60 mg prednisolone per day for 2 or 3 months. In both type I and type II, when possible, amiodarone should be withdrawn.[16]

Lithium and cytokines (interferon-αand interleukin-2) can also cause painless thyroiditis as a result of destruction of the gland and release of preformed thyroid hormone into circulation.[6,13] High-dose propranolol and methamphetamine use may cause inhibition of T4 to T3 conversion. Heparin may cause spurious T4 elevations.[6] Exogenous glucocorticoids and dopamine may cause a mild and transient decrease of TSH, which returns to normal once these medications are discontinued.[4]

The immune checkpoint inhibitors, ipilimumab and nivolumab, used in the treatment of melanoma, may cause thyroid autoimmunity with Graves ophthalmopathy or autoimmune thyroiditis. The thyroiditis may be either a permanent Hashimoto-type hypothyroidism or a transient, painless thyroiditis. In case studies, TPO antibodies and/or Tg antibodies were positive. Patients who undergo treatment with these medications should have baseline thyroid function studies and be monitored for new onset thyroid disease, especially during the first 3 months of treatment.[15,17]

PITUITARY OR HYPOTHALAMIC DISORDER

If the FT4 is also low, pituitary or hypothalamic disorder, also known as secondary (central) hypothyroidism, should be considered. Isolated central hypothyroidism is uncommon and usually presents with other pituitary hormone deficiencies including hypogonadism. Signs of hypogonadism include amenorrhea, impotence, and loss of body hair. These patients should undergo pituitary function testing and pituitary MRI.[1]

FACTITIOUS THYROID HORMONE INGESTION

Factitious thyroid hormone ingestion includes intentional, iatrogenic, and unintentional ingestion whether due to poisoning, pharmacy error, or consumption of supplements that contain thyroid extracts. Surreptitious use of thyroid hormone can be identified by absent goiter, low serum Tg level, decreased RAIU, and a disproportionately elevated T3 level.[6,11]

If the patient has previously been diagnosed with hypothyroidism and is currently taking levothyroxine, the dose should be adjusted and thyroid function tests repeated in 8 weeks.[1]

THYROID STORM

Thyroid storm is a rare, potentially life-threatening condition resulting from excessive circulating thyroid hormone from any cause. It may be caused by Graves disease, TA, TMG, excessive levothyroxine intake (intentional or unintentional), transient destructive thyroiditis due to virus, medications, autoimmunity, abrupt cessation of ATDs, or thyroid or nonthyroidal surgery in a patient with unrecognized or inadequately treated thyrotoxicosis or following RAI ablation.[3,6] It is characterized by systemic decompensation and high mortality if not immediately recognized and treated. Criteria include tachycardia, arrhythmias, congestive heart failure, hypotension, hyperpyrexia, agitation, delirium, psychosis, stupor, coma, nausea, vomiting, diarrhea, and hepatic failure. Treatment includes β-blockers, ATDs, inorganic iodine, steroids, aggressive cooling with acetaminophen and cooling blankets, volume resuscitation, respiratory support, and intensive care unit monitoring. Once ATDs have been started, administration of inorganic iodine (as potassium iodide oral solution, Lugol solution, or oral radiocontrast dye) will rapidly decrease T3 and T4 levels.[6]

TREATMENT OF GRAVES DISEASE

Treatment options for Graves disease include RAI treatment, ATDs, and surgical removal. All are effective and relatively safe.[6] Quality of life following treatment has been found to be the same in patients randomly allocated to one of these 3.[18] The decision should be made collaboratively between patient and treating clinician. This discussion should include a review of the logistics, benefits, expected recovery time, drawbacks, side effects, and cost.[6] Without treatment, up to 30% of patients will undergo remission.[19]

RADIOACTIVE IODINE

RAI treatment with ^{131}I is the therapy most preferred by US physicians, while European and Japanese physicians prefer ATDs and/or surgery. It has been used in the treatment of hyperthyroidism for 60 years. It is well tolerated, and complications, such as thyroid storm, are rare, except for those related to ophthalmopathy.[6]

RAI is preferred for women who plan to become pregnant in the intermediate (6 to 12 months) future, patients with comorbidities that increase surgical risk, and patients who have previously undergone neck surgery or external radiation treatment. Other reasons to consider RAI treatment include lack of access to a surgeon with high-volume experience and contraindications to ATD use. It is more desirable when patients prefer definitive, relatively rapid control of symptoms or avoidance of surgery or adverse effects of ATDs. Patients who choose RAI must understand the need for lifelong thyroid hormone replacement and be aware that resolution of symptoms may be lengthy.[6] It can take up to 12 weeks to achieve full effect.[4] RAI is not recommended in patients with moderate to severe active ophthalmopathy, because it may worsen thyroid eye disease. RAI is contraindicated in pregnant or breastfeeding patients or when patients plan to become pregnant within 4 to 6 months following treatment. RAI is also contraindicated when thyroid cancer is present or suspected, or patients are unable to comply with radiation safety guidelines.[6] Patients may not have been exposed to iodinated contrast or amiodarone in the 3 months before ablation.[4]

No special diet is required before RAI treatment, but patients should avoid sources of excessive iodine, which include iodine-containing multivitamins, seaweed, and kelp. A pregnancy test should be obtained within 48 hours of treatment in women with childbearing potential.[6]

Patients with severe symptoms or FT4 levels 2 to 3 times the upper limit of normal should be treated with β-blockers and/or ATDs, and medical treatment of comorbid conditions should be optimized before treatment with RAI.[6]

The amount given in a single dose should be adequate to make the patient hypothyroid. Ten to 15 mCi is generally sufficient; this quantity can also be calculated based on RAIU and gland size.[6]

Some patients will have anterior neck pain from radiation thyroiditis or worsening thyrotoxic symptoms as a result of leakage of preformed thyroid hormones from the damaged thyroid gland.[3]

Most patients have resolution of thyrotoxic symptoms at 4 to 8 weeks following treatment. Hypothyroidism occurs between 2 and 6 months after treatment. Initiation of thyroid hormone replacement should be based on thyroid function tests, symptoms, and physical examination and titrated based on FT4 levels. Thereafter, levels should be assessed annually. Conception should be postponed 4 to 6 months following RAI treatment to ensure stable levels of thyroid hormone levels on replacement.[6]

ANTITHYROID MEDICATIONS

ATDs include MMI and PTU. They inhibit thyroid peroxidase to block synthesis of T3 and T4.[4] They can be used long term or as a bridge to RAI ablation or surgery. Consider ATDs for patients with high likelihood of remission: patients, especially women, with mild disease, small goiters, and negative or low levels of TRAbs. ATDs are also appropriate for elderly patients, and patients with comorbidities that increase surgical risk or decrease life expectancy, who live in care facilities, or who may have difficulty following treatment recommendations after radiation. ATDs are the best choice for patients with Graves ophthalmopathy, and those who wish to avoid lifelong thyroid hormone replacement, surgery, or exposure to radioactivity. Patients beginning treatment with ATDs should be aware of potential adverse drug effects and the need for continued monitoring. Contraindications include previous known major adverse reactions to ATDs.[6]

ATDs control hyperthyroidism but do not cure Graves disease. They may have an immunosuppressive role, but their main effect is to reduce thyroid hormone and maintain euthyroid state while patients await spontaneous remission.[6,20]

MMI is preferred over PTU in all patients except pregnant women during the first trimester. PTU is used during the first trimester of pregnancy, in thyroid storm, and in patients with minor adverse reactions to MMI. Adverse drug effects include rash, agranulocytosis, and hepatic injury. Patients should be instructed to stop the medication and advise the provider of pruritic rash, jaundice, acholic stools or dark urine, arthralgias, abdominal pain, nausea, fatigue, fever, or pharyngitis. Agranulocytosis, vasculitis, and fulminant hepatic necrosis are rare, but more common in PTU than MMI; therefore, MMI is preferred over PTU.[6,21]

One should consider performing a baseline complete blood count and hepatic panel before initiating treatment with ATDs. Be aware that hyperthyroidism itself may cause mild liver function test abnormalities. In the event of febrile illness or pharyngitis, obtain a differential white blood cell count. If a patient develops agranulocytosis on MMI or PTU, use of the other agent is contraindicated because of cross-reactivity. Mild rashes may be managed with antihistamine therapy and continuation of the ATD.[6]

At the start of therapy with MMI, higher doses (10–40 mg daily) are recommended to achieve euthyroidism, after which the dose may be titrated to maintenance.[6,7] Maintenance doses are often 5 to 10 mg daily. MMI offers once-a-day dosing and reduced risk of severe adverse effects. PTU has a shorter duration of action and should be administered 2 or 3 times a day, starting with 50 to 150 mg at each dose. As clinical findings and thyroid function tests return to normal, reduce to a maintenance dose of 50 mg 2 or 3 times per day. Check TSH and FT4 levels every 4 to 8 weeks until the patient is euthyroid. Thereafter, evaluate the patient and laboratory test results every 2 to 3 months. TSH may remain suppressed for several months after starting therapy, and dose adjustment should be based on FT4 rather than TSH early in the course of treatment.[6]

After 12 to 18 months, MMI may be tapered or discontinued if the TSH remains normal. Measurement of TRAb levels help predict which patients can be weaned. Normal levels suggest a higher chance of remission. Check thyroid function tests every 1 to 3 months for 6 months to a year in order to identify relapse early. Instruct patients to contact the provider if symptoms of hyperthyroidism recur.[6]

Patients with normal serum TSH, FT4, and T3 for 1 year after discontinuation of ATD are considered to be in remission. In the United States, 20% to 30% of patients have durable remission. Remission rates are not improved by a course of ATDs longer than 18 months.[6,21] Lower rates of remission are seen in men, smokers, and those with large goiters.[6]

In patients who develop recurrent hyperthyroidism after a course of MMI, consider RAI ablation, thyroidectomy, or low-dose MMI again.[6]

In pregnancy, ATDs cross the placenta in small amounts and may cause fetal hypothyroidism. Low doses of PTU during the first trimester and MMI during second and third trimester is advisable. Doses should be just high enough to keep the mother's FT4 high-normal to slightly thyrotoxic. MMI is associated with cutis aplasia, and esophageal and choanal atresia in newborns, and therefore, should be avoided in the first trimester.[3,6]

THYROIDECTOMY

Surgery is appropriate for symptomatic compression due to large goiters, large nonfunctioning nodules, or when RAIU is low. It is preferred when malignancy is suspected (suspicious or indeterminate cytology) or when surgery is required anyway for coexisting hyperparathyroidism. Patients who want to become pregnant in the very near future (without sufficient time for thyroid hormone levels to become normal if RAI was chosen) or who have moderate to severe active Graves ophthalmopathy should choose surgery.[6]

Total or near-total thyroidectomy offers prompt and definitive control of hyperthyroidism and avoids exposure to radioactivity and the potential adverse effects of ATDs. It poses the risks inherent to surgery and requires lifelong thyroid replacement. Complications include transient or permanent hypocalcemia, temporary or permanent recurrent or superior laryngeal nerve injury, postoperative bleeding, and complications of anesthesia. Patients should be referred to a high-volume thyroid surgeon to avoid these surgical complications. Substantial comorbidity, such as cardiopulmonary disease, end-stage cancer, and other debilitating conditions, are contraindications to surgical treatment of Graves disease. When rapid control of hyperthyroidism is required and antithyroid medications cannot be used, surgery may be appropriate. Surgery should not be performed on pregnant patients during the first and third trimesters due to concerns about teratogenicity with anesthetic agents, increased risk of fetal loss, and preterm labor. If required during pregnancy, thyroidectomy is best performed at the end of the second trimester.[6]

Patients should be made euthyroid with MMI before surgery to prevent thyroid storm caused by the stress of surgery, anesthesia, and thyroid manipulation. Potassium iodine, given as 5 to 7 drops of Lugol's solution, should also be given 3 times daily for 10 days before surgery to decrease thyroid blood flow and reduce intraoperative blood loss. ATDs should be stopped at the time of surgery, and β-blockers should be weaned following surgery.[6]

When surgery is urgent, or patients are intolerant of ATDs, patients should be treated with corticosteroids preoperatively and β-blockers and potassium iodine immediately postoperatively.[6]

Following total thyroidectomy, patients should be started on levothyroxine at a weight-based dose (1.7 μg/kg) and TSH measured at 6 to 8 weeks postoperatively. Once stable and normal, TSH should be checked annually.[6]

Calcium or intact parathyroid hormone levels should be measured, and calcium and calcitriol should be supplemented based on results. Patients may be discharged from the hospital if they are asymptomatic and levels are 7.8 mg/dL or greater. Routine postoperative supplementation prevents the development of symptoms and allows for an earlier, safer discharge. Postoperative evaluation should be done at 1 or 2 weeks after discharge and supplementation continued based on test results.[6]

β-BLOCKERS

Symptomatic patients may benefit from treatment with β-blockers.[6] β-Blockers reduce heart rate, systolic blood pressure, muscle weakness, and tremor and improve irritability, emotional lability, and exercise intolerance.[3,6] Propranolol has the longest history of use for this purpose and is preferred in breastfeeding mothers. It may also block conversion of T4 to T3. Propranolol may be used at 10 to 40 mg 3 or 4 times a day. Atenolol is associated with the highest compliance given its once-a-day dosing option. Atenolol 25 to 100 mg may be given once or twice a day. Metoprolol, nadolol, and esmolol may also be used.[6] In addition to β-blockers, consider addressing myocardial ischemia, congestive heart failure, or atrial arrhythmias, if present. Patients with atrial fibrillation may require anticoagulation.[22]

SUMMARY

The appropriate screening test for thyroid dysfunction is serum TSH. A TSH within the normal range excludes primary thyroid disease. Other useful tests include FT4, T3, and serum Tg, TRAbs, TPO antibodies, and RAIU scan. Causes of low TSH include hyperthyroidism, thyrotoxicosis, TA, TMG, SH, thyroiditis, medications, pregnancy, hypothalamic or pituitary disease, overtreatment of hypothyroidism, surreptitious use of thyroid hormone, and nonthyroidal illness. Graves disease is the most common cause of hyperthyroidism. It can be treated with RAI, ATDs, or surgery. Secondary causes of thyroid dysfunction are relatively rare.

REFERENCES

1. Weetman AP. Investigating low thyroid stimulating hormone (TSH) level. BMJ 2013;347:f6842.
2. Hollowell JG, Staehling NW, Flanders WD, et al. Serum TSH, T(4), and thyroid antibodies in the United States population (1988 to 1994): National Health and Nutrition Examination Survey (NHANES III). J Clin Endocrinol Metab 2002;87(2):489–99.
3. Pearce EN. Diagnosis and management of thyrotoxicosis. BMJ 2006;332: 1369–73.
4. Kravets I. Hyperthyroidism: diagnosis and treatment. Am Fam Physician 2016; 93(5):363–70.
5. de los Santos ET, Starich GH, Mazzaferri EL. Sensitivity, specificity, and cost-effectiveness of the sensitive thyrotropin assay in the diagnosis of thyroid disease in ambulatory patients. Arch Intern Med 1989;149(3):526–32.
6. Bahn RS, Burch HB, Cooper DS, et al. Hyperthyroidism and other causes of thyrotoxicosis: management guidelines of the American Thyroid Association and American Association of Clinical Endocrinologists. Thyroid 2011;21(6): 593–646.
7. Castro RC, Gharib H. Thyroid disorders. In: Evidence-based endocrinology. 3rd edition. Philadelphia: Lippincott William and Wilkins; 2012.
8. US National Library of Medicine. Radioactive iodine uptake. MedlinePlus. Available at: https://www.nlm.nih.gov/medlineplus/ency/article/003689.htm. Accessed May 22, 2016.
9. US National Library of Medicine. Thyroid scan. MedlinePlus. Available at: https://www.nlm.nih.gov/medlineplus/ency/article/003829.htm. Accessed May 22, 2016.
10. Trzepacz PT, Klein I, Roberts M, et al. Graves' disease: an analysis of thyroid hormone levels and hyperthyroid signs and symptoms. Am J Med 1989;87(5): 558–61.

11. Walker P. Silent thyroiditis. Can Fam Physician 1984;30:1337–9.
12. Pearce EN, Farwell AP, Braverman LE. Thyroiditis. N Engl J Med 2003;328(26): 2646–55.
13. Collet TH, Gussekloo J, Bauer DC, et al. Subclinical hyperthyroidism and the risk of coronary heart disease and mortality. Arch Intern Med 2012;172(10):799–809.
14. Cooper DS, Biondi B. Subclinical thyroid disease. Lancet 2012;379:1142–54.
15. Min L, Vaidya A, Becker C. Thyroid autoimmunity and ophthalmopathy related to melanoma biological therapy. Eur J Endocrinol 2011;164:303–7.
16. Narayana SK, Woods DR, Boos CJ. Management of amiodarone-related thyroid problems. Ther Adv Endocrinol Metab 2011;2(3):115–26.
17. Ryder M, Callahan M, Postow MA, et al. Endocrine-related adverse events following ipilimumab in patients with advanced melanoma: a comprehensive retrospective review from a single institution. Endocr Relat Cancer 2014;21(2): 371–81.
18. Abraham-Nordling M, Wallin G, Lundell G, et al. Thyroid hormone state and quality of life at long-term follow-up after randomized treatment of Graves' disease. Eur J Endocrinol 2007;156:173–9.
19. Codaccioni JL, Orgiazzi J, Blanc P, et al. Lasting remissions in patients treated for Graves' hyperthyroidism with propranolol alone; a pattern of spontaneous evolution of the disease. J Clin Endocrinol Metab 1987;67(4):656–70.
20. Laurberg P. Remission of Graves' disease during anti-thyroid drug therapy. Time to reconsider the mechanism? Eur J Endocrinol 2006;155:783–6.
21. Abraham P, Avenell A, Park CM, et al. A systematic review of drug therapy for Graves' hyperthyroidism. Eur J Endocrinol 2005;153:489–98.
22. Ventrella S, Klein I. Beta-adrenergic receptor blocking drugs in the management of hyperthyroidism. Endocrinologist 1994;4(5):391.

Initial Evaluation and Workup of Thyroid Nodules in Adults

Christopher Sadler, MA, PA-C, CDE[a,b,*]

KEYWORDS

- Thyroid nodule • Thyroid cancer • Thyroid ultrasound • Hypoechoic
- Microcalcifications

KEY POINTS

- Most thyroid nodules encountered in clinical practice are benign; however, evaluation is needed to rule out thyroid cancer.
- Screening for risk factors—family history, childhood radiation exposure, or recent onset of voice hoarseness—can help identify individuals at higher risk for thyroid cancer.
- Physical examination findings that increase suspicion of malignancy include cervical lymphadenopathy, vocal cord paralysis, and a fixed, firm palpable nodule.
- Thyroid-stimulating hormone (TSH) testing is recommended for initial evaluation of thyroid nodules; suppressed TSH level can identify patients who need a radionuclide thyroid scan.
- High-risk ultrasound characteristics, such as nodules greater than 1 cm, solid consistency, hypoechoic echotexture, microcalcifications, or irregular borders, can help to identify potentially malignant nodules.

INTRODUCTION

Palpable thyroid nodules are discovered during routine examinations in approximately 5% of women and 1% of men in iodine-replete parts of the world.[1,2] Studies using high-resolution ultrasound (US) imaging have detected a prevalence of thyroid nodules in 19% to 68% of randomly selected individuals, with increased incidence in women and in the elderly.[3,4] The vast majority of thyroid nodules are benign; however, the clinical importance of thyroid nodules rests on excluding malignancy, which occurs in 7% to 15% of nodules depending on age, sex, and other risk factors for thyroid cancer.[5,6]

Disclosure Statement: C. Sadler is a full-time employee of AstraZeneca and holds AstraZeneca stock. The author reports no financial disclosures related to the topic of this article.
[a] Diabetes and Endocrine Associates, 9850 Genesee Ave #415, La Jolla, CA 92037, USA;
[b] AstraZeneca Pharmaceuticals LP, Medical Affairs Department, 1800 Concord Pike, Wilmington, DE 19897, USA
* Diabetes and Endocrine Associates, 9850 Genesee Ave #415, La Jolla, CA 92037, USA.
E-mail address: c.sadler@sbcglobal.net

Papillary and follicular cancers (differentiated thyroid cancers) comprise the majority (>90%) of all thyroid cancers. In 2014, it was estimated that there were 63,000 cases of newly diagnosed thyroid cancers,[7] compared with 37,200 cases diagnosed in 2009. The annual incidence of thyroid cancer has almost tripled from 1975 to 2009.[8] The majority of this is attributable to increased prevalence of papillary cancers. One study predicts that by 2019, papillary thyroid cancer will become the third most common cancer in women.[9]

In 2015, the American Thyroid Association (ATA) updated its guidelines for the management of adult patients with thyroid nodules and differentiated thyroid cancer.[10] This article references many of the recommendations from the guidelines with a primary focus on the initial workup and evaluation of thyroid nodules in adults. Primary care clinicians should be familiar with the evaluation of thyroid nodules and US characteristics that identify nodules at greater risk for malignancy so that appropriate referrals for diagnostic tests and specialists can be made in a timely manner.

THYROID NODULE DEFINITION AND GUIDING CLINICAL CONTEXT

Thyroid nodules are discrete lesions within the thyroid gland that are radiologically distinct from the surrounding thyroid parenchyma. A palpable abnormality on physical examination that does not have a corresponding radiographic abnormality does not meet the strict definition of a thyroid nodule.[11] Nodules that are nonpalpable and detected by thyroid US examination or other imaging studies are termed incidentally discovered nodules or "incidentalomas."[10] These nonpalpable incidentalomas have the same risk of cancer as palpable nodules of the same size.[12] Individuals with 1 palpable nodule found during a physical examination will have additional nodules found during a US examination 50% of the time.[13] In general, only nodules greater than 1 cm should be evaluated because they have a greater potential to be clinically significant cancers.[10] However, nodules that are less than 1 cm and have other suspicious features, such as surrounding lymphadenopathy and/or risk factors such as exposure to radiation or a family history of thyroid cancer, warrant further evaluation. There are very rare thyroid cancers that present as nodules less than 1 cm and do not exhibit the typical high-risk US or clinical features but still may cause significant morbidity and mortality. It is deemed that the cost–benefit ratio is unfavorable, and attempts to diagnose and treat all such small cancers will cause more harm than good.[10] This statement from the 2015 ATA thyroid nodule guidelines provides a good summary of the overarching clinical context: "In general, the guiding clinical strategy acknowledges that most thyroid nodules are low risk, and many thyroid cancers pose minimal risk to human health and can be effectively treated."[10]

INITIAL EVALUATION OF THYROID NODULES

A normal radionuclide examination will show even distribution of tracer throughout the thyroid gland (Fig. 1A). A low thyroid-stimulating hormone (TSH) level may be indicative of a hyperfunctioning nodule ("hot nodule"), which will reveal increased tracer uptake compared with surrounding thyroid tissue on a radionuclide scan (Fig. 1B) or a toxic multinodular goiter, which reveals patchy increased tracer uptake throughout the thyroid gland (Fig. 1C). Given that hyperfunctioning nodules have a very low risk for malignancy, no further workup for thyroid cancer is typically recommended. Hypofunctioning nodules show decreased tracer uptake compared with the surrounding thyroid tissue on a scan also referred to as a "cold nodule" (Fig. 1D). These cannot exclude thyroid cancers; however, the majority of nodules are hypofunctioning or "cold" on radionuclide scans and are not thyroid cancers.

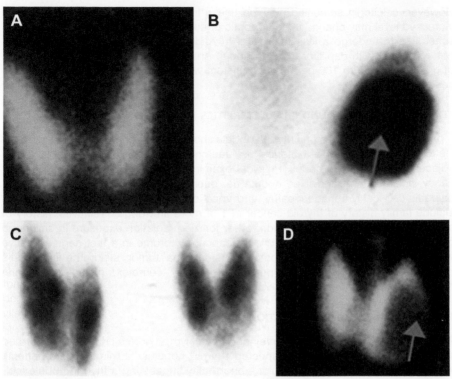

Fig. 1. Radionuclide examination of thyroid nodules. (*A*) Normal thyroid scan with uniform uptake of tracer throughout gland. (*B*) Hot nodule, increased tracer uptake concentrated in 1 area (*arrow*). (*C*) Patchy tracer uptake in a toxic multinodular goiter. (*D*) Cold nodule, reduced tracer uptake in nonfunctioning thyroid tissue (*arrow*).

Therefore, this is not a specific diagnostic examination and is not recommend in the initial workup in the absence of a suppressed TSH level.

This discrimination can be a helpful examination in select cases. For example, in a patient with Graves disease with a distinct nodule on US examination that is found to be "cold" or hypofunctioning on a radionuclide scan would increase the suspicion of a coexisting thyroid cancer and would warrant further evaluation. An elevated TSH level, even within the upper limit of the normal range, is associated with increased risk of malignancy.[14,15] Individuals with multiple distinct nodules on thyroid US examination do not have a reduced incidence of thyroid cancer as was once thought; therefore, each nodule should be evaluated based on US criteria, and high-risk nodules should be selected for further evaluation by fine needle aspiration (FNA).

OTHER SERUM MARKERS

The routine measurement of the serum thyroglobulin level is not recommended because this marker is increased in most forms of thyroid diseases and is insensitive and nonspecific for thyroid cancer.[10] It is, however, a useful cancer marker in patients who have undergone complete thyroidectomy for differentiated thyroid cancer.

There is insufficient evidence for recommending routine calcitonin screening, the serum marker for medullary thyroid cancer in patients with thyroid nodules.[10]

However, calcitonin screening may be useful in a subset of patients, because an increased level may change the diagnostic or surgical approach for a patient who is scheduled to undergo a less than total thyroidectomy or has suspicious cytology not consistent with papillary thyroid cancer. An unstimulated serum calcitonin level of greater than 50 to 100 pg/mL is consistent with a diagnosis of medullary thyroid cancer.[16]

CLINICAL AND ULTRASOUND CHARACTERISTICS AND THE RISK FOR MALIGNANCY

A patient with a diagnosis of a thyroid nodule should have a complete physical examination and assessment of historical risk factors focused on the thyroid gland and adjacent cervical lymph nodes. Physical examination findings suspicious for malignancy include a firm and fixed nodule (ie, does not freely move with swallowing), palpable cervical lymphadenopathy, and vocal cord paralysis. Historical risk factors include family history of thyroid cancer in 1 or more first-degree relatives, history of childhood head and neck irradiation, other ionizing radiation exposure in childhood or adolescence (eg, fallout), and thyroid cancer syndrome in a first-degree relative (eg, phosphatase and tensin homolog hamartoma tumor syndrome [Cowden's disease], familial adenomatous polyposis, Carney complex, multiple endocrine neoplasia 2 and, Werner syndrome/progeria).[17]

THYROID ULTRASOUND EXAMINATION

A thyroid US examination with survey of cervical lymph nodes should be performed in all patients with known or suspected thyroid nodules.[10] This includes patients with a nodular goiter or radiographic abnormality suggesting a thyroid nodule incidentally detected on another imaging study (MRI, computed tomography,[18] PET with F 18 fluorodeoxyglucose imaging uptake in thyroid, carotid US examination).[10] Important characteristics and US features of nodules as listed in the 2015 ATA guidelines[10] are shown in **Table 1**. The guidelines[10] arrange these US characteristics into 5 US patterns with associated risk of malignancy, which are shown in **Table 2**.

Thyroid US reports should include the location, size, number, and character of significant abnormalities, including measurement of nodules and focal abnormalities in 3 dimensions.[18] Unfortunately, some reports are of poor quality and do not give adequate details for risk assessment. An example of a poor report would be: "Enlarged thyroid gland with multiple nodules present bilaterally." In this example, there is no mention of the size, location, or characteristics of each nodule to determine if further evaluation is warranted. Additionally, there is no mention of whether there was an assessment of cervical lymph nodes.

Examples of US characteristics of thyroid nodules and their appearance on US examination, with associated risk for malignancy and indication for FNA are depicted in **Figs. 2–9**. High-risk US patterns include a solid hypoechoic nodule with interrupted rim calcification with soft tissue extrusion and a nodule with irregular margins and a suspicious cervical lymph node.

CERVICAL LYMPH NODE CHARACTERISTICS

Fig. 10 shows an US image of a normal-shaped lymph node, and **Fig. 11** shows an US image of an abnormal lymph node. Lymph node characteristics that increase the risk of malignancy[19] are the presence of microcalcifications, cystic aspect, peripheral vascularity, hyperechogenicity and round shape.

Table 1
Characteristics of nodules

Characteristic	Features
Size	Measured in 3 dimensions (depth, width, length)
Location	Right/left/isthmus Upper Mid Lower Anterior Posterior
Sonographic features	
Composition	Solid Cystic portion Spongiform
Echogenicity	Hypoechoic Isoechoic Hyperechoic
Margins	Regular Irregular
Type of calcifications	Micro Macro Rim Interrupted rim
Shape	Taller than wide in transverse view[a]
Extrathyroidal extension	Present Absent

[a] Increases risk of malignancy.

Adapted from Haugen Bryan R, Alexander Erik K, Bible Keith C, et al. 2015 American Thyroid Association Management guidelines for adult patients with thyroid nodules and differentiated thyroid cancer: the American Thyroid Association guidelines task force on thyroid nodules and differentiated thyroid cancer. Thyroid 2016;26(1):1–133.

FINE NEEDLE ASPIRATION

If it is determined that FNA is indicated based on the US characteristics and associated risk for malignancy, it can be performed using palpation. However, nodules that are poorly palpable, have a posterior location, or are partially cystic/solid are

Table 2
Sonographic patterns with associated risk of malignancy

Sonographic Pattern	Risk of Malignancy (%)
Benign	<1
Very low suspicion	<3
Low suspicion	5–10
Intermediate suspicion	10–20
High suspicion	>70–90

Data from Haugen Bryan R, Alexander Erik K, Bible Keith C, et al. 2015 American Thyroid Association Management guidelines for adult patients with thyroid nodules and differentiated thyroid cancer: the American Thyroid Association guidelines task force on thyroid nodules and differentiated thyroid cancer. Thyroid 2016;26(1):1–133.

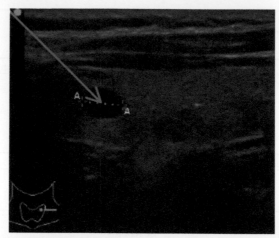

Fig. 2. Cystic nodule. The arrow tip is in the center of a purely cystic nodule (benign sonographic pattern), which are typically benign, carry a risk of malignance of less than 1%, and typically do not meet criteria for fine needle aspiration (FNA). However, if a cyst is large and symptomatic, aspiration to drain fluid and relieve symptoms is appropriate. Some centers use ethanol ablation of the cyst after drainage to reduce risk of recurrence. If FNA is performed, the cystic fluid should be sent for cytologic evaluation. (*Data from* Haugen Bryan R, Alexander Erik K, Bible Keith C, et al. 2015 American Thyroid Association Management guidelines for adult patients with thyroid nodules and differentiated thyroid cancer: the American Thyroid Association guidelines task force on thyroid nodules and differentiated thyroid cancer. Thyroid 2016;26(1):1–133.)

best suited for FNA under US guidance. Studies have shown that US-guided needle placement during FNA of thyroid nodules reduces the incidence of nondiagnostic and false-negative cytology.[20,21] In partially cystic and solid nodules, the solid portion of the nodule would be targeted for sampling by FNA under US guidance.

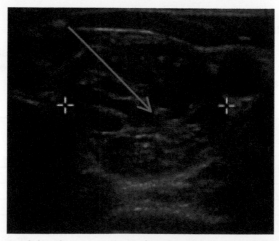

Fig. 3. Spongiform nodule. The arrow tip is placed in the center of a spongiform nodule. Spongiform appearance refers to the presence of multiple microcystic areas comprising more than 50% of the nodule's volume. These nodules have a less than 3% risk for malignancy (very low suspicion sonographic pattern). Given the higher likelihood of benign cytology, fine needle aspiration is only recommended for nodules 2.0 cm or greater in size.

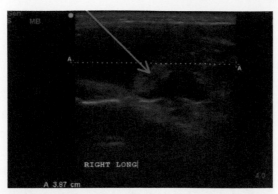

Fig. 4. Partially cystic nodule. The arrow tip is touching a solid portion of a mostly cystic nodule. Partially cystic or "mixed nodule" falls into the "very low suspicion" sonographic pattern category with a less than 3% risk of malignancy. If there are eccentric solid portions within the nodule, the risk of malignancy increases to 5% to 10% (low suspicion sonographic pattern). Fine needle aspiration (FNA) should be considered for nodules 2.0 cm or greater in size, with FNA sampling directed toward the solid portions of the nodule under ultrasound guidance.

FINE NEEDLE ASPIRATION CYTOLOGY

The Bethesda System for Reporting Thyroid Cytopathology is widely accepted as the standard for reporting thyroid cytopathology.[22,23] There are 6 diagnostic categories to this system, and there is an estimation of cancer risk based on literature review and expert opinion. The diagnostic categories are nondiagnostic or unsatisfactory, benign, atypia of undetermined significance or follicular lesion of undetermined significance, follicular neoplasm or suspicious for follicular neoplasm, suspicious for malignancy, and malignant.

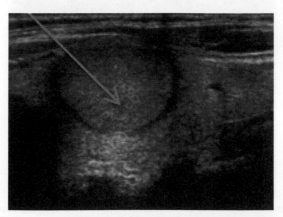

Fig. 5. Solid isoechoic or hyperechoic nodules with regular margins. The arrow tip is in the center of a solid isoechoic nodule; the nodule has a similar echogenicity to the surrounding normal thyroid tissue. A hyperechoic nodule would be brighter than the surrounding tissue. Notice that this nodule is well demarcated by a surrounding halo with regular margins. These nodules carry a risk of malignancy of 5% to 10% (low risk sonographic pattern); fine needle aspiration is recommended for nodules 1.5 cm or greater in size.

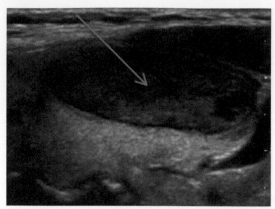

Fig. 6. Solid hypoechoic nodule. The arrow tip is in the central portion of this large mostly solid hypoechoic nodule with regular margins. This type of nodule has a risk for malignancy of 10% to 20% (intermediate risk sonographic pattern), and nodules greater than 1.0 cm in size are indicated for fine needle aspiration.

Nondiagnostic or Unsatisfactory

Results from an FNA cytology should generally be repeated, because the actual risk of malignancy in nodules within this category that were surgically excised ranges from 9% to 32%.[24] Patients should have the FNA repeated with US guidance and onsite cytology if available to determine the adequacy of the sample. Repeat FNA should ideally be performed no sooner than 3 months after the initial FNA to prevent false-positive interpretation owing to biopsy-induced reactive/reparative changes.[25]

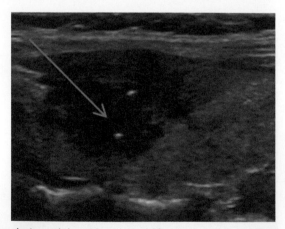

Fig. 7. Solid hypoechoic nodule with microcalcifications and irregular margins. The arrow tip is near the center of this solid hypoechoic nodule. Of note is the irregular shape of the margins of this nodule; the 2 bright spots within the nodule are microcalcifications. This nodule has a greater than 70% to 90% risk of malignancy (high suspicion sonographic pattern). Fine needle aspiration is recommended for nodules 1.0 cm or greater in size, although smaller nodules could be sampled if there are other suspicious features, such as abnormal cervical lymph nodes.

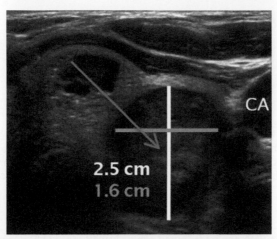

Fig. 8. Solid hypoechoic nodule – taller than wide in the transverse view. The arrow tip is near the center of this solid hypoechoic nodule, which is taller in the transverse view (2.5 cm) compared with the width (1.6 cm) in the same view. This nodule has a greater than 70% to 90% risk of malignancy (high suspicion sonographic pattern). Fine needle aspiration is indicated for nodules 1.0 cm or greater in size.

Nodules with repeated nondiagnostic samples without high-suspicion US patterns should be followed closely and may not require surgical removal. A high-suspicion US pattern nodule with repeated nondiagnostic samples that is growing during ongoing US examinations or in a patient with clinical risk factors for malignancy should be considered for surgical removal.

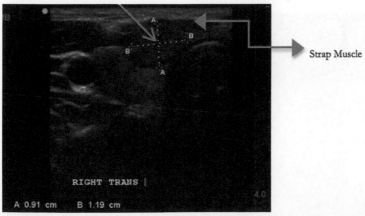

Fig. 9. Nodule with extracapsular invasion. The arrow tip is within this solid hypoechoic nodule near the isthmus of the thyroid gland and is extending beyond the thyroid capsule into the strap muscle superiorly. Of note is that there is no clear demarcation between the nodule and the strap muscle, signifying invasion of the nodule into the strap muscle. This nodule has a greater than 70% to 90% risk of malignancy (high suspicion sonographic pattern). Fine needle aspiration (FNA) is recommended for nodules 1.0 cm or greater in size. Based on FNA and surgical pathology samples, this nodule proved to be papillary thyroid cancer.

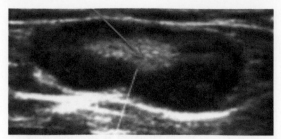

Fig. 10. Normally shaped lymph node. Benign-appearing lymph nodes are typically twice as wide as tall in the transverse view with a distinct hilar line running down the center of the node. The arrow tip points to the hilar line of a normal-appearing cervical lymph node in transverse view.

Benign

Benign cytology on FNA can be followed clinically with repeat US examinations as indicated by the US pattern, with closer follow-up of higher risk US pattern nodules. There is a small risk (1%–3%) of a false-negative benign cytology.[26–31] However, long-term studies are quite reassuring. In 1369 patients with 2010 cytologically benign nodules followed for 8.5 years, only 18 malignancies were detected, with no deaths caused by thyroid cancer in this cohort.[32] The absence of a high death rate from most thyroid cancers is something that should be emphasized to patients and their families.

Two benign cytologies from the same nodule virtually rules out malignancy[26–30] and continued surveillance of these nodules by US examination is not recommended.[10] Occasionally, a benign nodule on cytology may be recommended for surgical removal owing to other factors such as patient preference, symptoms, and/or being of excessive size (>4 cm). There is still unclear evidence to determine if these larger nodules pose a higher risk of malignancy.[10]

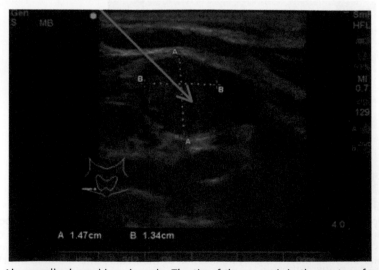

A 1.47cm   B 1.34cm

Fig. 11. Abnormally shaped lymph node. The tip of the arrow is in the center of an abnormally rounded cervical lymph node in the right lower neck just inferior and lateral to the right thyroid lobe in a patient with metastatic papillary thyroid cancer. Of note is that the lymph node is rounded in appearance in the transverse view and the hilar line is absent.

Atypia of Undetermined Significance or Follicular Lesion of Undetermined Significance Cytology

This an indeterminate category that is not clearly benign or malignant. This diagnostic category leaves clinicians in a quandary as to whether to continue to follow the nodule clinically or send the patient for surgical excision. The US pattern can help to guide clinical decision making in that a high-risk pattern is more likely to be malignant and may cause the clinician to lean toward surgical intervention, as would significant risk factors such as radiation exposure or positive family history.

Recently, the use of molecular testing of FNA samples from nodules with these indeterminate cytologies has been studied[33] and is currently used in some clinics. The purpose of these molecular tests is to better inform the clinician regarding the probability of malignancy in a given cytologically indeterminate nodule. Three molecular panels are currently available for clinical use: (1) a 7-gene panel of genetic mutations and rearrangements,[34] (2) a 167-gene expression classifier,[35] and (3) immunohistochemical stains.[36] According to expert opinion and analysis,[10] there is currently no single optimal molecular test that can definitively rule out malignancy in all cases of indeterminate cytology. Long-term data on clinical utility of these markers are still lacking. This is a rapidly evolving field, and ongoing research may still produce new useful markers or validate current markers for guiding clinical decision making. Patients considering molecular testing should be counseled on the potential benefits and limitations as well as about possible uncertainties in the clinical implications of results.[10]

Follicular Neoplasm or Suspicious for Follicular Neoplasm

For this category, FNA cytology is typically managed by the long-established standard of care of surgical excision because the diagnosis can only be made definitively by examining the margins of the nodule after removal. Supplementing the risk assessment with the US features of the nodule and molecular testing can postpone or obviate the need for going directly to surgery; however, close follow-up of the patient is warranted.

Suspicious for Malignancy and Malignant

For this category, FNA cytology will typically recommend these nodules for surgical excision. However, there are clinical factors that may change this recommendation. For example, surgery may not be the best course of action for a clearly malignant nodule in a patient who is a poor surgical candidate owing to comorbid conditions, or if the patient is likely to succumb to another illness before the thyroid cancer becomes clinically relevant.

FOLLOW-UP OF NODULES WITH BENIGN CYTOLOGY ON ULTRASOUND-GUIDED FINE NEEDLE ASPIRATION

Follow-up of nodules with benign US-guided FNA cytology should be based on the US risk category of the given nodule. The 2015 ATA guidelines[10] recommend the following:

A. *Nodules with a high suspicion US pattern:* repeat US examination and US-guided FNA within 12 months.
B. *Nodules with a low to intermediate suspicion US pattern:* repeat US examination at 12 to 24 months. If there is US evidence of growth (20% increase in ≥2 nodule dimensions with a minimal increase of 2 mm or >50% change in volume) or development of new suspicious US features, repeat FNA or continue observation with repeat US examinations; repeat FNA in case of continued growth.

C. *Nodules with a very low suspicion US pattern (including spongiform nodules):* the usefulness of surveillance US and assessment of nodule growth as an indicator for repeat FNA to detect a missed malignancy is limited. If US examination is repeated, it should be done after more than 24 months.

D. If a nodule has undergone repeat US-guided FNA with a second benign cytology result, US surveillance for this nodule for continued risk of malignancy is no longer indicated.

SUMMARY

Primary care clinicians familiar with the current standard of care for the evaluation and management of thyroid nodules can more effectively advise their patients and refer them to appropriate specialty care. Appropriate evaluation of a suspected thyroid nodule begins with assessment of thyroid function based on the TSH level. Low TSH values should be further evaluated by radionuclide examination to rule out a hyperfunctioning nodule, which is virtually always benign. If the TSH is not suppressed, high-resolution US examination of the thyroid and cervical lymph nodes is the preferred method for detection and characterization of a risk of a particular nodule for malignancy based on specific US features. These features can guide the clinician on the need for an FNA procedure as well as the extent of ongoing surveillance, if any. FNA cytology along with clinical and historical findings, can guide the specialist clinician regarding the need for surgery and the extent of surgery. The clinician should reassure patients and families that the outcome of therapy for the vast majority of thyroid nodules is excellent.

REFERENCES

1. Vander JB, Gaston EA, Dawber TR. The significance of nontoxic thyroid nodules. final report of a 15-year study of the incidence of thyroid malignancy. Ann Intern Med 1968;69:537–40.
2. Tunbridge WM, Evered DC, Hall R, et al. The spectrum of thyroid disease in a community: the Whickham survey. Clin Endocrinol (Oxf) 1977;7:481–93.
3. Tan GH, Gharib H. Thyroid incidentalomas: management approaches to nonpalpable nodules discovered incidentally on thyroid imaging. Ann Intern Med 1997; 126:226–31.
4. Guth S, Theune U, Aberle J, et al. Very high prevalence of thyroid nodules detected by high frequency (13 MHz) ultrasound examination. Eur J Clin Invest 2009;39:699–706.
5. Hegedus L. Clinical practice. The thyroid nodule. N Engl J Med 2004;351:1764–71.
6. Mandel SJ. A 64-year-old woman with a thyroid nodule. JAMA 2004;292:2632–42.
7. Siegel R, Ma J, Zou Z, et al. Cancer statistics, 2014. CA Cancer J Clin 2014;64: 9–29.
8. Davies L, Welch HG. Current thyroid cancer trends in the United States. JAMA Otolaryngol Head Neck Surg 2014;140:317–22.
9. Aschebrook-Kilfoy B, Schechter RB, Shih YC, et al. The clinical and economic burden of a sustained increase in thyroid cancer incidence. Cancer Epidemiol Biomarkers Prev 2013;2:1252–9.
10. Haugen Bryan R, Alexander Erik K, Bible Keith C, et al. 2015 American Thyroid Association Management guidelines for adult patients with thyroid nodules and differentiated thyroid cancer: the American Thyroid Association Guidelines task force on thyroid nodules and differentiated thyroid Cancer. Thyroid 2016;26(1): 1–133.

11. Marqusee E, Benson CB, Frates MC, et al. Usefulness of ultrasonography in the management of nodular thyroid disease. Ann Intern Med 2000;133:696–700.
12. Hagag P, Strauss S, Weiss M. Role of ultrasound-guided fine-needle aspiration biopsy in evaluation of nonpalpable thyroid nodules. Thyroid 1998;8:989–95.
13. Jarlov AE, Nygaard B, Hegedus L, et al. Observer variation in the clinical and laboratory evaluation of patients with thyroid dysfunction and goiter. Thyroid 1998;8: 393–8.
14. Boelaert K, Horacek J, Holder RL, et al. Serum thyrotropin concentration as a novel predictor of malignancy in thyroid nodules investigated by fine-needle aspiration. J Clin Endocrinol Metab 2006;91:4295–301.
15. Haymart MR, Repplinger DJ, Leverson GE, et al. Higher serum thyroid stimulating hormone level in thyroid nodule patients is associated with greater risks of differentiated thyroid cancer and advanced tumor stage. J Clin Endocrinol Metab 2008;93:809–14.
16. Gagel RF, Hoff AO, Cote GE. Medullary thyroid carcinoma. In: Braverman L, Utiger R, editors. Werner and Ingbar's the thyroid. Philadelphia: Lippincott Williams and Wilkins; 2005. p. 967–88.
17. Richards ML. Familial syndromes associated with thyroid cancer in the era of personalized medicine. Thyroid 2010;20:707–13.
18. American Institute of Ultrasound in Medicine. AIUM Practice Parameter for the performance of a Thyroid and Parathyroid Ultrasound Examination. Laurel, MD: American Institute of Ultrasound in Medicine; 2013.
19. Leenhardt L, Erdogan MF, Hegedus L, et al. 2013 European Thyroid Association guidelines for cervical ultrasound scan and ultrasound-guided techniques in the postoperative management of patients with thyroid cancer. Eur Thyroid J 2013;2: 147–59.
20. Danese D, Sciacchitano S, Farsetti A, et al. Diagnostic accuracy of conventional versus sonography-guided fine-needle aspiration biopsy of thyroid nodules. Thyroid 1998;8:15–21.
21. Carmeci C, Jeffrey RB, McDougall IR, et al. Ultrasound-guided fine-needle aspiration biopsy of thyroid masses. Thyroid 1998;8:283–9.
22. Baloch ZW, LiVolsi VA, Asa SL, et al. Diagnostic terminology and morphologic criteria for cytologic diagnosis of thyroid lesions: a synopsis of the National Cancer Institute Thyroid Fine-Needle Aspiration State of the Science Conference. Diagn Cytopathol 2008;36:425–37.
23. Crippa S, Mazzucchelli L, Cibas ES, et al. The Bethesda System for reporting thyroid fine-needle aspiration specimens. Am J Clin Pathol 2010;134:343–4.
24. Bongiovanni M, Spitale A, Faquin WC, et al. The Bethesda System for Reporting Thyroid Cytopathology: a meta-analysis. Acta Cytol 2012;56:333–9.
25. Layfield LJ, Abrams J, Cochand-Priollet B, et al. Post-thyroid FNA testing and treatment options: a synopsis of the National Cancer Institute Thyroid Fine Needle Aspiration State of the Science Conference. Diagn Cytopathol 2008;36:442–8.
26. Chehade JM, Silverberg AB, Kim J, et al. Role of repeated fine-needle aspiration of thyroid nodules with benign cytologic features. Endocr Pract 2001;7:237–43.
27. Orlandi A, Puscar A, Capriata E, et al. Repeated fine-needle aspiration of the thyroid in benign nodular thyroid disease: critical evaluation of long-term follow-up. Thyroid 2005;15:274–8.
28. Oertel YC, Miyahara-Felipe L, Mendoza MG, et al. Value of repeated fine needle aspirations of the thyroid: an analysis of over ten thousand FNAs. Thyroid 2007; 17:1061–6.

29. Erdogan MF, Kamel N, Aras D, et al. Value of re-aspirations in benign nodular thyroid disease. Thyroid 1998;8:1087–90.
30. Illouz F, Rodien P, Saint-Andre JP, et al. Usefulness of repeated fine-needle cytology in the follow-up of non-operated thyroid nodules. Eur J Endocrinol 2007;156:303–8.
31. Tee YY, Lowe AJ, Brand CA, et al. Fine needle aspiration may miss a third of all malignancy in palpable thyroid nodules: a comprehensive literature review. Ann Surg 2007;246:714–20.
32. Nou E, Kwong N, Alexander LK, et al. Determination of the optimal time interval for repeat evaluate after a benign thyroid nodule aspiration. J Clin Endocrinol Metab 2014;99:510–6.
33. Xing M, Haugen BR, Schlumberger M. Progress in molecular-based management of differentiated thyroid cancer. Lancet 2013;381:1058–69.
34. Nikiforov YE, Ohori NP, Hodak SP, et al. Impact of mutational testing on the diagnosis and management of patients with cytologically indeterminate thyroid nodules: a prospective analysis of 1056 FNA samples. J Clin Endocrinol Metab 2011;96:3390–7.
35. Alexander EK, Kennedy GC, Baloch ZW, et al. Preoperative diagnosis of benign thyroid nodules with indeterminate cytology. N Engl J Med 2012;367:705–15.
36. Bartolazzi A, Orlandi F, Saggiorato E, et al. Galectin-3-expression analysis in the surgical selection of follicular thyroid nodules with indeterminate fine-needle aspiration cytology: a prospective multicentre study. Lancet Oncol 2008;9:543–9.

Obesity: "Can the Battle Be Won?"

Shannon McShea, PA-C, MSPAS, CNSC

KEYWORDS

- Obesity • Weight loss pharmacotherapy • Bariatric surgery • Nutritional deficiencies

KEY POINTS

- Overweight and obesity affects more than 60% of the adult population in the United States.
- Obesity is associated with an increased rate of diabetes mellitus type 2, obstructive sleep apnea, dyslipidemia, fatty liver disease, hypertension, degenerative joint disease, and some cancers.
- The US Food and Drug Administration has approved 4 medications in the last few years to help with weight loss: phentermine-topiramate (Qsymia), lorcaserin (Belviq), bupropion-naltrexone (Contrave), and liraglutide (Saxenda).
- Bariatric surgery is an effective tool for weight loss and treatment of comorbid conditions. All bariatric procedures have potential risks and complications. Postsurgery patients need long-term vitamin supplementation and nutritional monitoring.

DEFINING OVERWEIGHT AND OBESITY

Since 1985, the National Institutes of Health (NIH) has been using the body mass index (BMI) to define overweight and obesity. In 1998, the BMI cutoffs for overweight and obesity were modified to those that are in current use (**Table 1**).[1] The BMI is calculated by dividing a person's weight in kilograms by the squared height in meters (kg/m^2). The BMI is used to classify overweight and obesity and to estimate relative risk of disease compared with normal weight. The BMI is not diagnostic of health status, rather, it is a screening tool, and is not without flaw. For example, many lean athletes may have a high BMI because of high muscle mass. According to BMI criteria, a BMI less than $18.5 \ kg/m^2$ is underweight, 18.5 to $24.9 \ kg/m^2$ is normal weight, 25 to $29.9 \ kg/m^2$ is overweight, 30 to $34.9 \ kg/m^2$ is obesity (class I), 35 to $39.9 \ kg/m^2$ is obesity (class II), and greater than $40 \ kg/m^2$ is severe obesity (class III). The severe obesity class is sometimes further divided into superobese (BMI, $50–59.9 \ kg/m^2$) and super-super–obese (BMI, $>60 \ kg/m^2$). To calculate the BMI, a free tool is available at the National Heart, Lung, and Blood Institute (NHLBI) Web site: http://www.nhlbi.nih.gov/health/educational/lose_wt/BMI/bmicalc.htm.

Disclosure: Received honorarium from Takeda pharmaceutical.
Department of Nutrition and Weight Management, Geisinger Medical Center, 100 North Academy Avenue, MC 21-11, Danville, PA 17821, USA
E-mail address: smmcshea@geisinger.edu

Physician Assist Clin 2 (2017) 87–106
http://dx.doi.org/10.1016/j.cpha.2016.08.008
2405-7991/17/

Table 1
Classification of overweight and obesity by body mass index, waist circumference, and associated disease risk.

			Waist circumference in inches	
	BMI (kg/m^2)	Obesity Class	Men ≤40 in. Women ≤35 in.	Men >40 in. Women >35 in.
Underweight	<18.5		—	—
Normal[a]	18.5–24.9		—	—
Overweight	25.0–29.9		Increased	High
Obesity	30.0–34.9	I	High	Very high
	35.0–39.9	II	Very high	Very high
Extreme obesity	≥40	III	Extremely high	Extremely high

[a] Increased waist circumference can also be a marker for increased risk even in persons of normal weight.
From National Institutes of Health, National Heart, Lung, and Blood Institute in cooperation with the National Institute of Diabetes and Digestive and Kidney Diseases. Clinical guidelines on the identification, evaluation, and treatment of overweight and obesity in adults: the evidence report. NIH Publication no. 98-4083. Available from: http://www.nhlbi.nih.gov/guidelines/obesity/ob_gdlns.pdf.

In addition to the BMI, accessing fat distribution is an important factor. Abdominal circumference measurement gives more information for determining health risk than BMI alone. For consistency, waist measurements should be taken at the level of the ileac crest (**Fig. 1**).[2] The apple (android) and pear (gynoid) shapes refer to extra weight in the abdominal (visceral) area versus the hip/buttock/thigh (subcutaneous), respectively. Visceral weight is associated with greater risk of cardiometabolic disease.[3] The risk of cardiometabolic diseases (coronary heart disease, hypertension, and type-2 diabetes) is increased, even in people with a normal BMI, if the waist circumference is larger than 40 inches for men or 35 inches for women.

OBESITY TRENDS

The prevalence of overweight and obesity in the United States is staggering. The 2011 to 2012 National Health and Nutrition Examination Survey (NHANES) reports 69% of US adults are overweight, 35% have a BMI greater than 30 kg/m^2, 14.5% have a BMI greater than 35 kg/m^2, and 6.4% have a BMI greater than 40 kg/m^2 (**Fig. 2**).[4] The NHANES data for overweight, obesity, and severe obesity from 1960 to 2012 are depicted in **Fig. 3**. One can see the steep increase in obesity starting in 1980 and continuing through 2005. During the last 12 to 15 years, the prevalence of obesity has not changed significantly.[5] However, the prevalence of *severe* obesity (BMI >40 kg/m^2) is still increasing.[6]

CONSEQUENCES OF OBESITY

Obesity affects most every organ system in the body (**Fig. 4**).[7] With a greater BMI comes increased risk for cardiometabolic diseases, such as hypertension, dyslipidemia, cardiovascular disease (CVD), hypercoagulability causing blood clots, and type 2 diabetes. Certain cancers are associated with obesity, including breast, colon, uterine, pancreatic, kidney, and prostate. Risk of obstructive sleep apnea, degenerative joint disease, gallbladder disease, nonalcoholic fatty liver disease, pseudotumor cerebri, gastric reflux, and infertility are all increased with excess weight. Mental health disorders, including depression, anxiety, and body image disorders, are seen with obesity.[8]

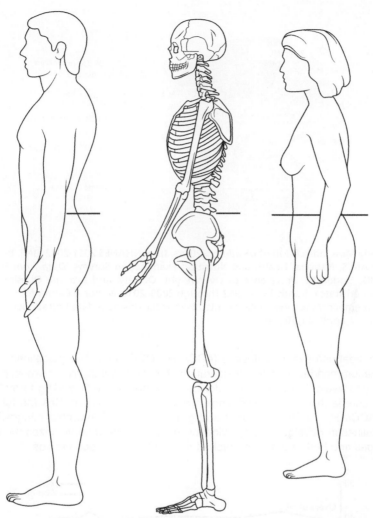

Fig. 1. Measuring tape position for waist (abdominal) circumference. (*From* Obesity Education Initiative Electronic Textbook. Available at: http://www.nhlbi.nih.gov/health-pro/guidelines/current/obesity-guidelines/e_textbook/txgd/4142.htm. Accessed April 14, 2016.)

Obesity pervades all aspects of life, including socioeconomic status, social discrimination, and social stigmatization.

GUIDELINES FOR MANAGEMENT OF OVERWEIGHT AND OBESITY IN ADULTS

Overweight and obesity have a role in most chronic diseases managed in the primary care setting. In 2013 the American Heart Association (AHA), American College of Cardiology (ACC), and The Obesity Society developed and published a clinical practice guideline titled Expert panel report: Guidelines (2013) for the management of overweight and obesity in adults.[9] The recommendations outlined in the guidelines were based on current research and experts/panel members' responses to 5 clinical questions. The recommendations were graded by both the NHLBI format (**Table 2**) and the American College of Cardiology/American Heart Association Class of

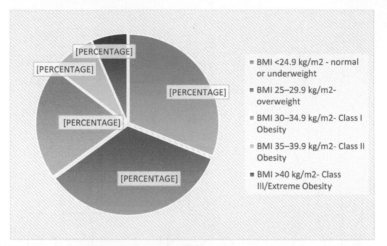

Fig. 2. Body Mass Index (BMI) of US adults >20 yrs. from NHANES 2011-2012. BMI, body mass index; NHANES, National Health and Nutrition Examination Surveys. *Data from* Fryar CD, Carroll MD, Ogden CL. Prevalence of Overweight, Obesity, and Extreme Obesity Among Adults: United States, Trends 1960–1962 Through 2009–2010. National Center for Health Statistics. September 2012. Available at: http://www.cdc.gov/nchs/data/hestat/obesity_adult_09_10/obesity_adult_09_10.htm.

Recommendation/Level of Evidence (ACC/AHA COR/LOE). The guidelines address lifestyle recommendations and considerations for bariatric surgery; however, pharmacotherapy for weight loss was not addressed. Although the 2 grading formats have different criteria, the recommendations are in overall alignment. See the full article for the ACC/AHA COR/LOE format and grades at http://www.nhlbi.nih.gov/health-pro/guidelines/in-develop/obesity-evidence-review .**Table 3** summarizes the recommendations and NHLBI grade for each of the guideline's 5 focus topics.

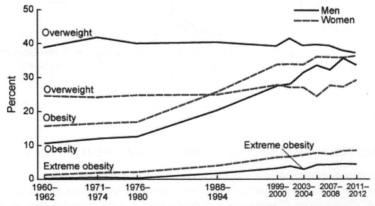

Fig. 3. Trends in adult overweight, obesity, and extreme obesity among men and women 20 to 74 years: United States, selected years 1960 to 1962 through 2011 to 2012. *Data from* Fryar CD, Carroll MD, Ogden CL. Prevalence of overweight, obesity, and extreme obesity among adults: United States, trends 1960–1962 through 2009–2010. National Center for Health Statistics. 2012. Available at: http://www.cdc.gov/nchs/data/hestat/obesity_adult_09_10/obesity_adult_09_10.htm.)

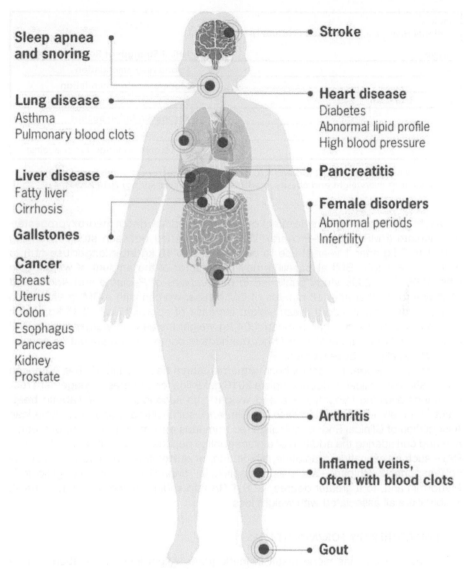

Sleep apnea and snoring

Stroke

Lung disease
Asthma
Pulmonary blood clots

Heart disease
Diabetes
Abnormal lipid profile
High blood pressure

Liver disease
Fatty liver
Cirrhosis

Pancreatitis

Female disorders
Abnormal periods
Infertility

Gallstones

Cancer
Breast
Uterus
Colon
Esophagus
Pancreas
Kidney
Prostate

Arthritis

Inflamed veins, often with blood clots

Gout

Fig. 4. Medical complications of obesity. (*Adapted from* Yale University Rudd Center for Food Policy and Obesity CDC- Vital Signs –Medical Complications of Obesity. Available at: http://www.cdc.gov/vitalsigns/AdultObesity/infographic.html. Accessed April, 14, 2016.)

MEDICATIONS ASSOCIATED WITH WEIGHT GAIN

In addition to encouraging weight loss by lifestyle modifications, it is important for providers to consider the potential impact that medications can have on weight. Medications that act centrally have the potential to alter the hypothalamic appetite and satiety center. Certain antidepressants, antipsychotics, antidiabetics, anticonvulsants, antihistamines, antihypertensives, and glucocorticoids are linked with weight gain (**Box 1**).[10]

Table 2	
National Heart, Lung and Blood Institute grade system	
Grade	NHLBI Strength of Recommendation
A	Strong recommendation
B	Moderate recommendation
C	Weak recommendation
D	Recommendation against
E	Expert opinion
N	No recommendation for or against

Data from Jensen MD, Ryan DH, Donato KA, et al. Expert panel report: guidelines (2013) for the management of overweight and obesity in adults. Obesity (Silver Spring) 2014;22:S41–410.

Weight gain is a common side effect of the contraceptive, depot medroxyprogesterone acetate (DMPA)/(Depo-Provera). Weight gain varied between studies, ranging from 1 to 2 kg after 1 year of use to between 4 and 10 kg after longer use of 3 to 5 years.[11] Patients' BMI at baseline may be a factor of the amount of weight gain with DMPA.[12] A 2006 study published in *the Archives of Pediatric and Adolescent Medicine* found that after 18 months of DMPA use, women with a BMI greater than 30 kg/m² at baseline had a mean weight increase of approximately 9.45 kg, which was significantly higher than a mean 4.04 kg weight increase in women with a BMI less than 25 kg/m² at baseline.[12] Other methods of contraception should be considered, especially in obese women.

In the last decade, the antidiabetic armamentarium has expanded. The American Association of Clinical Endocrinologists 2016 guideline for diabetes management recommends avoiding hypoglycemia and weight gain secondary to antidiabetic treatment.[13] In an effort to decrease insulin and sulfonylurea dose, the American Association of Clinical Endocrinologists recommends maximizing the dose of metformin and considering the addition of a glucagonlike peptide-1 receptor agonist (GLP-1 RA)—such as exenatide, liraglutide, albiglutide, or dulaglutide—or a sodium-glucose cotransporter-2 inhibitor—such as canagliflozin, dapagliflozin, or empagliflozin.[13] Metformin and, to a greater degree, GLP-1 RA and sodium-glucose cotransporter-2 inhibitor are all associated with weight loss.[13]

PHARMACOTHERAPY FOR WEIGHT LOSS

If lifestyle interventions alone result in inadequate weight loss, medication can be added as an adjunctive treatment. Medication use is indicated for patients with a BMI greater than 30 kg/m² or for a BMI greater than 27 kg/m² with weight-related comorbidities. The US Food and Drug Administration (FDA) approved multiple new drugs over the last 4 years. However, many primary care providers are hesitant to prescribe them, in part because of the litigious history of weight loss medications. Fenfluramine was half of the famous phentermine/fenfluramine combination, otherwise known as *Phen-Fen*. Fenfluramine and the chemically related drug dexfenfluramine were recalled by the FDA in 1997 because of risks of valvular heart disease and primary pulmonary hypertension. A little more than a decade later in 2010, sibutramine (Meridia), a serotonin–norepinephrine reuptake inhibitor, was also taken off market because of increased cardiac events.[14]

The current FDA-approved medications for weight loss include phentermine, orlistat, lorcaserin, phentermine/topiramate, bupropion/naltrexone, and liraglutide.

Table 3
Summary of recommendation for obesity

Recommendation	NHLBI Grade
Identifying patients who need to lose weight	
Measure height and weight and calculated BMI at least annually.	E
Use BMI classification for overweight and obese to identify adults who may be at elevated risk of CVD. Use BMI for obesity to identify adults who may be at elevated risk of mortality from all causes.	A
Advise overweight and obese adults that the greater the BMI, the greater the risk of CVD, type 2 diabetes, and all-cause mortality.	A
Measure waist circumference at annual visits or more frequently in overweight and obese adults. Advise adults that the greater the waist circumference, the greater the risk of CVD, type 2 diabetes, and all-cause mortality. Increased risk with waist >35 inches for women and >40 inches for men.	E
Matching treatment benefits with risk profiles (effect of body weight reduction on risk factors for CVD, events, morbidity, and mortality)	
• Counsel overweight and obese adults with cardiovascular risk factor (high blood pressure, hyperlipidemia, and hyperglycemia) that lifestyle changes that produce even modest, sustained weight loss of 3%–5% is likely to result in clinically meaningful health benefits. Greater weight losses produce greater benefits. ○ Sustained weight loss of 3%–5% is likely to result in clinically meaningful reduction in triglycerides, blood glucose, hemoglobin A1c, and the risk of type 2 diabetes. ○ Greater amounts of weight loss will reduce blood pressure, improve low-density lipoprotein cholesterol and high-density lipoprotein cholesterol, and reduce the need for medications to control blood pressure, blood glucose, and lipids and further reduce triglycerides and blood glucose.	A
Diets for weight loss (dietary strategies for weight loss)	
• Prescribe a diet to achieve reduced calorie intake for obese or overweight individuals who would benefit from weight loss as part of a comprehensive lifestyle intervention. Any one of the following methods can be used to reduce food and calorie intake. ○ Prescribe 1200–1500 kcal/d for women and 1500–1800 kcal/d for men (kilocalorie levels are usually adjusted for the individual's body weight) ○ Prescribe a 500-kcal/d or 750-kcal/d energy deficit *or* ○ Prescribe one of the evidence-based diets that restricts certain food types (such as high-carbohydrate foods, low-fiber foods, or high-fat foods) to create an energy deficit by reduced food intake.	A
Prescribe a calorie-restricted diet for obese and overweight individuals who would benefit from weight loss, based on the patient's preferences and health status, and preferably refer to a nutrition professional for counseling.	A
Lifestyle intervention and counseling (comprehensive lifestyle intervention)	
Advise overweight and obese individuals who would benefit from weight loss to participate for ≥6 months in a comprehensive lifestyle program that assists participants in adhering to a lower-calorie diet and in increasing physical activity through the use of behavioral strategies.	A
Prescribe on-site, high-intensity (ie, ≥14 sessions in 6 months) comprehensive weight loss interventions provided in individual or group sessions by a trained interventionist.	A
Electronically delivered weight loss programs (including by telephone) that include personalized feedback from a trained interventionist can be prescribed for weight loss but may result in smaller weight loss than face-to-face interventions.	B

(*continued on next page*)

Table 3 (continued)	
Recommendation	**NHLBI Grade**
Some commercial bases that provide a comprehensive lifestyle intervention can be prescribed as an option for weight loss, provided there is peer-reviewed published evidence of their safety and efficacy.	B
Use a very low-calorie diet (defined as <800 kcal/d) only in limited circumstances and only when provided by trained practitioners in a medical care setting in which medical monitoring and high-intensity lifestyle intervention can be provided. Medical supervision is required because of the rapid rate of weight loss and potential for health complications.	A
Advise overweight and obese individuals who have lost weight to participate long term (≥1 year) in a comprehensive weight loss maintenance program. For weight loss maintenance, prescribe face-to-face or telephone-delivered weight loss maintenance programs that provide regular contact (monthly or more frequently) with a trained interventionist who helps participants engage in high levels of physical activity (ie, 200–300 min/wk), monitor body weight regularly (ie, weekly or more frequently), and consume a reduced-calorie diet (needed to maintain lower body weight).	A
Selecting patients for bariatric surgical treatment for obesity (bariatric surgical treatment for obesity)	
Advise adults with a BMI ≥40 kg/m² or BMI ≥35 kg/m² with obesity-related comorbid conditions who are motivated to lose weight and who have not responded to behavioral treatment with or without pharmacotherapy with sufficient weight loss to achieve targeted health outcome goals that bariatric surgery may be an appropriate option to improve health and offer referral to an experienced bariatric surgeon for consultation and evaluation.	A
For individuals with a BMI <35 kg/m², there is insufficient evidence to recommend for or against undergoing bariatric surgical procedures.	N
Advise patients that choice of a specific bariatric surgical procedure may be affected by patient factors, including age, severity of obesity/BMI, obesity-related comorbid conditions, other operative risk factors, risk of short- and long-term complications, behavioral and psychosocial factors, and patient tolerance for risk, as well as provider factors (surgeon and facility).	E

Adapted from Jensen MD, Ryan DH, Donato KA, et al. Expert panel report: guidelines (2013) for the management of overweight and obesity in adults. Obesity (Silver Spring) 2014;22:S41–410.

Table 4 lists each medication, the mechanism of action, the year of FDA approval, the contraindications for use, and the potential side effects. The mean weight loss reported for each medication is the amount seen in excess of placebo.[15] For example, a mean weight loss of 5 lb would be recorded if the patient on placebo lost 10 lb and the patient taking the drug lost 15 lb.

Phentermine is approved for short-term therapy (≤3 months), whereas all others are indicated for chronic/long-term use. Phentermine, lorcaserin, and phentermine/topiramate are all schedule IV controlled substances. Phentermine is a psychostimulant and has potential for misuse. Lorcaserin earned the schedule IV designation, because some patients reported hallucinations, euphoria, and "positive subjective responses" during drug trials, when given in supratherapeutic doses.[16] Orlistat, bupropion/naltrexone, and liraglutide are not controlled substances.

In addition to the information provided in **Table 5**, the following are other considerations for weight loss medication use. With chronic orlistat use, patients are at risk for

Box 1
Pharmacotherapy associated with weight gain
• Antipsychotics   ○ Clozapine, olanzapine, risperidone
• Antidepressants   ○ Paroxetine, mirtazapine, amitriptyline, imipramine
• Antidiabetics   ○ Insulin, sulfonylurea, thiazolidinedione
• Anticonvulsants   ○ Valproate, gabapentin, pregabalin
• Antihistamines   ○ Cyproheptadine, hydroxyzine
• Antihypertensive   ○ Beta blockers
• Glucocorticoids
• Progestin

deficiencies of the fat-soluble vitamins A, D, E, and K. The provider should recommend a complete multivitamin daily. In 2010, case reports of severe liver injury associated with orlistat use prompted the FDA to add a new warning to the product label.[17]

The efficacy of weight loss medications vary among individuals. Some patients are considered responders, whereas others are not. A nonresponder is defined as an individual that loses less than 5% of initial body weight after 12 weeks on the maximal dose of medication (4% with liraglutide).[18,19] Medication should be discontinued or an alternative option should be considered in nonresponders, as it is unlikely that meaningful weight loss will be achieved and sustained with continued treatment.[16,20,21]

Topiramate is a pregnancy category D (only use if benefits outweigh risks). Craniofacial birth defects have been reported.[20] Phentermine/topiramate, like all antiobesity medications, are pregnancy category X (risks outweigh any benefit).[16–19] According to the product insert, a negative pregnancy test should obtained in all women of childbearing age before starting phentermine/topiramate and monthly thereafter.[18] A provider must use caution when using topiramate in a patient with a history of kidney stones. Topiramate can promote kidney stone formation by reducing urinary citrate excretion and increasing urine pH levels. Topiramate should not be taken in combination with other drugs that inhibit carbonic anhydrase (such as zonisamide, acetazolamide, or methazolamide). Concurrent use of ketogenic diets and inadequate hydration can also increase the risk of stone formation.[21]

Liraglutide is a long-acting GLP-1 RA that was FDA approved in 2010 for the treatment of diabetes under the brand name Victoza. Further studies on patients without diabetes found significant weight loss as well.[22] When formulated as a weight loss medication, liraglutide (Saxenda) was given at 3.0 mg subcutaneously daily versus the target dose of 1.8 mg subcutaneously daily for diabetes management.

BARIATRIC SURGERY

The NIH criteria for candidate selection for bariatric surgery have been in place since 1991. Surgery can be offered to individuals with a BMI $\geq$40 kg/m^2 or a BMI $\geq$35 kg/m^2 with obesity-related comorbidities who attempted at least 6 months of a medically

Table 4
Comparison of medication for weight loss

Drug (Generic)	Dosage	Mechanism of Action	Weight Loss Above Diet and Lifestyle Alone Mean Weight Loss, % or kg[a]; Duration of Clinical Studies	FDA Drug Approval Date	Common Side Effects	Contraindications
Short-term use (3 mo)						
Phentermine resin	Adipex P (37.5 mg) 37.5 mg/d Ionamin (30 mg) 30–37.5 mg/d	Norepinephrine-releasing agent	3.6 kg (7.9 lb); 2–24 wk	1960s	Headache Elevated BP Elevated HR Insomnia Dry mouth Constipation Anxiety Cardiovascular Palpitation, tachycardia, elevated BP, ischemic events Central nervous system Overstimulation, restlessness, dizziness, euphoria, dysphoria, tremor, headache, psychosis Gastrointestinal Unpleasant taste, diarrhea, other gastrointestinal disturbances Allergic Urticaria Endocrine Impotence, changes in libido	Anxiety disorders (agitated states) History of heart disease Uncontrolled hypertension Seizure MAOIs Pregnancy and breastfeeding Hyperthyroidism Glaucoma History of drug abuse Sympathomimetic amines
Diethylpropion	Tenuate (75 mg) 75 mg/d	Norepinephrine-releasing agents	3.0 kg (6.6 lb); 6–52 wk	1960s	See Phentermine resin	See Phentermine resin

Chronic weight management

	Dose	Mechanism	Weight loss	Year	Side effects	Contraindications
Liraglutide	3.0 mg injectable	GLP-1 agonist	5.8 kg (12.8 lb); 1 y[11,12]	2014	Nausea Vomiting Pancreatitis	Medullary thyroid cancer history Multiple endocrine neoplasia type 2 history
Lorcaserin (10 mg)	10 mg twice a day	5HT2c receptor agonist	3.6 kg (7.9 lb), 3.6%; 1 y	2012	Headache Nausea Dry mouth Dizziness Fatigue Constipation	Pregnancy and breastfeeding use with caution SSRI SNRI/MAOI St John's wort Triptans Buproprion Dextromethorphan
Naltrexone/bupropion (NB)	32 mg/360 mg	Reuptake inhibitor of dopamine and norepinephrine (B) and opioid antagonist (N)	4.8%; 1 y[13]	2014	Nausea Constipation Headache Vomiting Dizziness	Uncontrolled hypertension, seizure disorders Anorexia nervosa or bulimia Drug or alcohol withdrawal MAOIs
Orlistat prescription (120 mg)	120 mg 3 times a day	Pancreatic and gastric lipase inhibitor	2.9–3.4 kg (6.5–7.5 lb), 2.9%–3.4%; 1 y	1999	Decreased absorption of fat-soluble vitamins Steatorrhrea Oily spotting Flatulence with discharge Fecal urgency Oily evacuation Increased defecation Fecal incontinence	Cyclosporine (taken 2 h before or after orlistat dose) Chronic malabsorption syndrome Pregnancy and breastfeeding Cholestasis Levothyroxine Warfarin Antiepileptic drugs

(continued on next page)

Table 4
(continued)

Drug (Generic)	Dosage	Mechanism of Action	Weight Loss Above Diet and Lifestyle Alone Mean Weight Loss, % or kg[a]; Duration of Clinical Studies	FDA Drug Approval Date	Common Side Effects	Contraindications
Orlistat over-the-counter (60 mg)	60–120 mg 3 times a day	Pancreatic and gastric lipase inhibitor	2.9–3.4 kg (6.5–7.5 lb), 2.9%–3.4%; 1 y	1999	See Orlistat prescription	See Orlistat prescription
Phentermine (P)/topiramate (T)	3.75 mg P/23 mg T ER every day (starting dose) 7.5 mg P/46 mg T ER daily (recommended dose) 11.25 mg P/69 mg T ER daily 15 mg P/92 mg T ER daily (high dose)	GABA receptor modulation (T) plus norepinephrine-releasing agent (P)	6.6 kg (14.5 lb) (recommended dose), 6.6% 8.6 kg (18.9 lb) (high dose), 8.6%; 1 y	2012	Insomnia Dry mouth Constipation Paresthesia Dizziness Dysgeusia	Pregnancy and breastfeeding Hyperthyroidism Glaucoma MAOIs Sympathomimetic amines

Abbreviations: BP, blood pressure; ER, extended release; HTN, hypertension; MAOI, monoamine oxidase inhibitor; selective, serotonin reuptake inhibitor; SNRI, serotonin-norepinephrine reuptake inhibitor; SSRI, selective serotonin reuptake inhibitors.

[a] Mean weight loss in excess of placebo as % initial body weight or mean kilogram weight loss over placebo.

Adapted from Apovian CM, Aronne LJ. The 2013 American Heart Association/American College of Cardiology/the obesity society guideline for the management of overweight and obesity in adults what is new about diet, drugs, and surgery for obesity? Circulation 2015;132:1589–90; with permission of the Endocrine Society.

Table 5
Vitamin and micronutrient recommendations for patients after metabolic surgery

	LAGB	VSG/RYGB	BPD/DS
Complete multivitamin-mineral supplement[a]	1 daily	2 daily	2 daily
Calcium citrate (total daily mg given in divided dose)	1200–1500 mg	1200–1500 mg	1200 mg–1500 mg
Vitamin D3[b]	3000 IU	3000 IU	3000 IU
Vitamin B12	MVI sufficient	As needed to maintain blood levels	As needed to maintain blood levels
Iron	If indicated to satisfy NRV if dietary intake plus routine supplement insufficient	45–60 mg (from multivitamin + additional supplements)	45–60 mg (from multivitamin + additional supplements)
Vitamin A			10,000 IU daily
Vitamin K			300 µg daily[c]

Further variation to the basic supplement recommendation is required to maintain nutritional status if dietary intake plus routine supplements is insufficient, and for pregnancy planning.

Separate iron and calcium supplements by at least 2 hours to enhance absorption.

Abbreviations: MVI, multivitamin; NRV, nutrient reference value.

[a] Containing 100% of daily value for at least two-thirds of nutrients, with a minimum of 18 mg iron and 400 g folic acid. Each serving should have thiamin, copper, selenium, and zinc.

[b] Titrate dose to therapeutic level greater than 30 ng/mL.

[c] Use caution with patients on warfarin therapy.

Data from Mechanisk JI, Youdim A, Jones DB, et al. AACE/TOS/ASMBS clinical practice guidelines for the perioperative nutritional, metabolic, and nonsurgical support of the bariatric surgery patient – 2013 update: cosponsored by American Association of Clinical Endocrinologists, The Obesity Society, and America Society for Metabolic & Bariatric Surgery. Obesity 2013;21:S1–27; and Aills L, Blankenship J, Buffington C, et al. ASMBS allied health nutritional guidelines for the surgical weight loss patient. Surg Obes Relat Dis 2008;4(5 Suppl):S73–108.

supervised weight loss program.[23] Most insurances follow the basic NIH criteria, but many have additional requirements and some have an exclusion to bariatric surgery.

The number of bariatric operations in the United States increased from 13,386 in 1998 to 220,000 in 2008.[24] Still, only 1% of the qualifying patients have surgery each year.[25] Surgery has become safer with mortality rates comparable to those of routine general surgical procedures such as laparoscopic cholecystectomy or fundoplication.[26] Many obesity-related medical conditions improve with weight loss (**Box 2**).[27]

SURGICAL PROCEDURES

In the United States, the roux-en-Y gastric bypass (RYGB) and vertical sleeve gastrectomy (VSG) are now the 2 most common bariatric procedures performed. Other procedures that have waxed and waned in popularity over the years include the

---

Box 2
Obesity-related comorbidities improved with weight loss

- Improved mortality (suggested by nonrandomized studies)
- Major cardiovascular event rates (myocardial infarction, stroke, and cardiovascular)
- Type 2 diabetes
- Nephropathy related to diabetes
- Type 2 diabetes prevention
- Hypertension
- Dyslipidemia
- Hyperuricemia
- Obstructive sleep apnea
- Obesity hypoventilation
- Nonalcoholic fatty liver disease and nonalcoholic steatohepatitis
- Degenerative joint disease (osteoarthritis of weight-bearing joints)
- General physical functioning and exercise capacity
- Recovery and rehabilitation following joint surgery
- Hirsutism
- Intertrigo and candidiasis
- Wound healing
- Polycystic ovarian disease
- Improved fertility (female and male)
- Regulation of menstrual cycle
- Reduction in overall cancer risk and mortality
- Quality-of-life health measures
- Cognitive function (improvement in learning and memory)
- Urinary incontinence

Data from Ding S, McKenzie T, Vernon AH, et al. Bariatric surgery. In: Jameson JL, De Groot JL, editors. Endocrinology: adult and pediatric. 7th edition. Philadelphia: Elsevier/Saunders; 2016. 479–90. Chapter 27.

laparoscopic adjustable gastric band (LAGB) and the biliopancreatic diversion (BPD), with or without the duodenal switch (BPD/DS). The bariatric surgeries are illustrated in **Figs. 4** and **5**.[28] The RYGB involves the creation of a small gastric pouch (about 1 ounce) that is connected to a segment of jejunum, which has been transected at 30 to 75 cm distal from the ligament of Treitz, to form a roux-en-Y limb. The excluded biliopancreatic limb is reattached approximately 75 to 150 cm distal to the gastrojejunostomy. Therefore, ingested food bypasses most of the stomach, the entire duodenum, and a small segment of the jejunum.[28]

LAGB involves placing a silicone ring with an inflatable inner tube around the upper stomach. The inner tube is connected to a subcutaneous port in the abdomen. The port is used to inject or withdraw saline to adjust the band diameter. Originally, the VSG was performed in higher-risk patients as a step to a staged BPD. The restrictive component led to weight loss that allowed the subsequent bowel bypass to be safer. Because of the success seen in some patients, the VSG has become a primary procedure. In the VSG, a vertical cut is made in the stomach, removing 75% of the stomach.[28]

The BPD involves a horizontal gastrectomy, leaving behind 200 to 500 mL of stomach, which is anastomosed to the small intestine, 250 cm from the ileocecal valve. The excluded biliopancreatic limb is anastomosed to the ileum, 50 cm from the ileocecal valve. Digestion takes place in the 50-cm common channel, where digestive

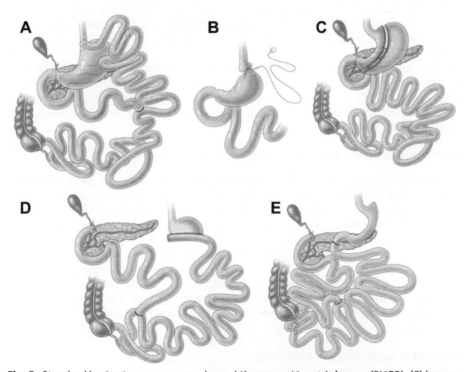

Fig. 5. Standard bariatric surgery procedures. (*A*) roux-en-Y gastric bypass (RYGB). (*B*) laparoscopic adjustable gastric banding (LAGB). (*C*) laparoscopic sleeve gastrectomy (LSG). (*D*) biliopancreatic diversion (BPD) and (*E*) BPD with duodenal switch[25]. *From* Bradley D, Magkos F, Klein S. Effects of bariatric surgery on glucose homeostasis and type 2 Ddabetes. Gastroenterology 2012;143:897–912.

secretions from the biliopancreatic limb mix with the ingested food delivered by the alimentary limb. BPD with duodenal switch involves constructing a 150- to 200-mL volume vertical sleeve gastrectomy with preservation of the pylorus and formation of a duodenal-ileal anastomosis. The excluded biliopancreatic limb is anastomosed to the ileum, 100 cm from the ileocecal valve, where digestive secretions and nutrients mix. These latter 2 procedures cause considerable malabsorption.[28]

SURGICAL COMPLICATIONS

All surgeries have perioperative risks, such as infection, thrombotic events, and anesthesia complications. Bariatric surgery has both early and late complications associated with each procedure. Early complications of bariatric surgery include anastomotic leaks and gastrointestinal bleeding.[28] Late complications include anastomotic ulcers, anastomotic strictures, and bowel obstruction. The risk of gastrojejunal ulceration is increased with tobacco and nonsteroidal anti-inflammatory drug use. Internal hernias occur from the openings created in the mesentery during the RYGB procedure. If undiagnosed, life-threatening bowel strangulation and necrosis can occur.[28]

Dumping syndrome occurs in individuals with the RYGB with the ingestion of concentrated sweets. The presence of high-osmolality food in the small intestine causes a fluid shift from the intravascular to enteric intraluminal space. Early dumping syndrome occurs within a half hour of eating and symptoms include nausea, abdominal pain, diarrhea, bloating, flushing, and tachycardia. Late dumping syndrome is caused by a hyperinsulinemia response to sugar intake. Low blood sugar symptoms (weak, diaphoresis, and shakiness) occur 2 to 3 hours after a meal.[28]

Weight regain after surgery can be caused by a combination of reasons, including behavioral (dietary indiscretions, lack of physical activity), mental health disorders, hormonal/metabolic changes, or surgical/anatomic issues. A gastrogastric fistula can occur after an RYGB. An abnormal connection is formed between the gastric pouch and the remnant/old stomach.[28]

NUTRITIONAL CONSEQUENCES OF WEIGHT-LOSS SURGERY

Nutritional deficiencies are observed after bariatric surgery. In RYGB, BPD, and BPD/DS, the proximal small bowel is bypassed, leading to significantly reduced absorption of vitamin B12, iron, calcium, vitamin D, copper, and zinc. Patients with a BPD or BPD/DS have a higher rate of fat-soluble vitamin deficiencies and protein malnutrition.[29] Iron deficiency is common, especially in menstruating women. Parenteral replacement may be necessary, as oral iron supplementation is often insufficient. Calcium and vitamin D supplementation must be encouraged, as metabolic bone disease is a common complication if supplements are neglected.[29] Calcium citrate is the preferred calcium supplement, as it is the most bioavailable calcium salt in a low acidic environment.[30] See **Table 5** for the recommended vitamin and mineral supplements after bariatric surgery.[31]

LONG-TERM NUTRITIONAL MONITORING

After bariatric surgery it is essential to monitor blood chemistries and screen for nutritional deficiencies. The recommended laboratory studies for each procedure are reviewed in **Table.6**.[32]

Table 6
Recommended blood tests (mo postsurgery)

	VSG	RYGB	BPD/DS
Chemistry panel	3, 6, 12 + A	3, 6, 12 + A	3, 6, 12 + A
Vitamin B1	3, 6, 12 + A	3, 6, 12 + A	3, 6, 12 + A
Vitamin B12	6, 12 + A	6, 12 + A	6, 12 + A
Vitamin A	—	6, 12 + A	6, 12 + A
Vitamin K	—	12 + A	12 + A
Vitamin D	12 + A	6, 12 + A	6, 12 + A
Iron	12 + A	3, 6, 12 + A	3, 6, 12 + A
Zinc	12 + A	6, 12 + A	6, 12 + A
Copper	—	12 + A	12 + A
Calcium	6, 12 + A	6, 12 + A	6, 12 + A
iPTH	12 + A	12 + A	12 + A
Albumin	12 + A	6, 12 + A	6, 12 + A

Abbreviations: A, annually; iPTH, intact parathyroid hormone.
 * Frequency may vary based on clinical indications.
 Data from Stein J, Stier C, Raab H, et al. Review article: the nutritional and pharmacologic consequences of obesity surgery. Aliment Pharmacol Ther 2014;40:582–609.

NUTRITIONAL EMERGENCY

Thiamin (vitamin B1) deficiency is truly a medical emergency. The body has a small reserve of thiamin. Vomiting after any bariatric surgery can deplete thiamin quickly. Untreated thiamin deficiency can lead to Wernicke's encephalitis, pontine stroke, long-term physical disability, or even death. Thiamine, intravenous or intramuscular, should be given immediately. See **Box 3** for symptoms of and treatment for thiamin deficiency.[29]

Box 3
Thiamin deficiency

• Can occur with prolonged vomiting after any bariatric surgery procedure.

• Do not wait for thiamin levels to return, as irreversible neurologic damage can occur.

Signs and Symptoms

• Ataxia, nystagmus

• Symmetric motor and sensory neuropathy with pain, paresthesia, loss of reflexes

• Irritability, muscle cramps, blurry vision, weakness, tripping over one's toes, unable to get out of tub

Treatment

• Intravenous or intramuscular thiamin, 100 mg immediately, (before any intravenous dextrose) x 7 days

• Oral supplement of thiamin, 50 to 100 mg daily, once tolerating diet

SUMMARY

In the last 30 years, the rate of obesity has doubled.[4] Obesity is caused by a complex interaction of environmental, social, economic, and behavioral factors along with genetic susceptibility. Likewise, the treatment plan needs to be multifactorial. Lifestyle/behavioral changes must be the foundation. Medication can be a helpful adjunct for some patients. Bariatric surgery remains the most effective tool for weight loss, weight maintenance, and resolution or mediation or obesity-related disease. Albeit, with potential short- and long-term complications.

Obesity has an obvious impact on the individual level, from physical health to overall quality of life. However, the ripple effect expands over the society as a whole. The obese have increased medical costs, decreased work productivity, and increased disability.[33] The economic burden on the health care system is great, especially on the tax-funded programs of Medicare and Medicaid.[34] Obesity has become a worldwide issue, coined *globesity*. Most of the world's population lives in countries in which now overweight and obesity kill more people than underweight.[35]

Prevention of obesity and early intervention in the treatment of obesity is imperative. Focusing on the family unit, in addition to the individual, is helpful in building support and teaching children healthier lifestyles. Multiple initiatives target communities, schools, and workplace for the prevention of obesity, ranging from increasing access to farmers markets to community development for safer walking/bike paths. Many resources are available through the Centers for Disease Control's Division of Nutrition, Physical Activity, and Obesity website http://www.cdc.gov/nccdphp/dnpao/state-local-programs/index.html.

REFERENCES

1. National Institutes of Health, National Heart, Lung, and Blood Institute. Clinical guidelines on the identification, and treatment of overweight and obesity in adults: the evidence report. no. 98-4083. Bethesda, MD: NIH Publication; 1998. Available at: http://www.nhlbi.nih.gov/files/docs/guidelines/ob_gdlns.pdf.
2. Obesity Education Initiative Electronic Textbook. Available at: http://www.nhlbi.nih.gov/healthpro/guidelines/current/obesity-guidelines/e_textbook/txgd/4142.htm. Accessed April 14, 2016.
3. Chan JM, Rimm EB, Colditz GA, et al. Obesity, fat distribution, and weight gain as risk factors for clinical diabetes in men. Diabetes Care 1994;17(9):961–9.
4. Fryar CD, Carroll MD, Ogden CL. Prevalence of overweight, obesity, and extreme obesity among adults: United States, trends 1960–1962 through 2009–2010. Atlanta, GA: National Center for Health Statistics; 2012. Available at: http://www.cdc.gov/nchs/data/hestat/obesity_adult_09_10/obesity_adult_09_10.htm.
5. Flegal KM, Carroll MD, Kit BK, et al. prevalence of obesity and trends in the distribution of body mass index among US adults, 1999-2010. JAMA 2012;307(5):491–7.
6. Sturm R, Hattori A. Morbid obesity rates continue to rise rapidly in the US. Int J Obes (Lond) 2013;37(6):889–91.
7. CDC- Vital Signs –Medical Complications of Obesity. Image (Adapted from Yale University Rudd Center for Food Policy and Obesity). Available at: http://www.cdc.gov/vitalsigns/AdultObesity/infographic.html. Accessed April, 14, 2016.
8. CDC-Division of Nutrition, Physical Activity, and Obesity, National Center for Chronic Disease Prevention and Health Promotion. Available at: http://www.cdc.gov/obesity/adult/causes.html Accessed April 14, 2016.
9. American College of Cardiology/American Heart Association Task Force on Practice Guidelines, Obesity Expert Panel, 2013. Expert panel report: Guidelines

(2013) for the management of overweight and obesity in adults. Obesity (Silver Spring) 2014;22:S41–410.

10. Kohlstadt I. Medications as modifiable contributors to weight gain. Medscape 2010. Available at: http://www.medscape.com/viewarticle/718977. Accessed April 14, 2016.

11. Bahamondes L, Del Castillo S, Tabares G, et al. Comparison of weight increase in users of depot medroxyprogesterone acetate and copper IUD up to 5 years. Contraception 2001;64(4):223–5. Available at: http://dx.doi.org/10.1016/S0010-7824(01)00255-4.

12. Bonny AE, Ziegler J, Harvey R, et al. Weight gain in obese and nonobese adolescent girls initiating depot medroxyprogesterone, oral contraceptive pills, or no hormonal contraceptive method. Arch Pediatr Adolesc Med 2006;160(1):40–5.

13. Garber A, Abrahamson M, Barzilay J, et al. Consensus statement by the American Association of Clinical Endocrinologists and American College of Endocrinology on the comprehensive type 2 diabetes management algorithm – 2016 executive summary. Endocr Pract 2016;22:84–113. Available at: https://www.aace.com/sites/all/files/diabetes-algorithm-executive-summary.pdf. Accessed April 14, 2016.

14. Astrup A. Drug Management of Obesity — Efficacy versus Safety. N Engl J Med 2010;363:288–90.

15. Apovian CM, Aronne LJ. The 2013 American Heart Association/American College of Cardiology/The Obesity Society Guideline for the Management of Overweight and Obesity in Adults What Is New About Diet, Drugs, and Surgery for Obesity? Circulation 2015;132:1586–91.

16. Belviq [package insert]. Available at: http://www.belviq.com/documents/Belviq_Prescribing_Information.pdf. Accessed April 14, 2016.

17. FDA Drug Safety Communication: Completed safety review of Xenical/Alli (orlistat) and severe liver injury. Available at: http://www.fda.gov/Drugs/DrugSafety/PostmarketDrugSafetyInformationforPatientsandProviders/ucm213038.htm. Accessed April 14, 2016.

18. Qsymia [package insert]. Available at: http://www.accessdata.fda.gov/drugsatfda_docs/label/2012/022580s000lbl.pdf. Accessed April 14, 2016.

19. Saxenda [package insert]. Available at: http://www.novo-pi.com/Saxenda.pdf. Accessed April 14, 2016.

20. Qsymia-FDA prescribing information, side effects, and uses. Available at: http://www.drugs.com/pro/qsymia.html. Accessed April 14, 2016.

21. Gazewood JD, Barry K. Phentermine/Topiramate (Qsymia) for Chronic Weight Management. Am Fam Physician 2014;90(8):576–8. Available at: http://www.aafp.org/afp/2014/1015/p576.html. Accessed April 14, 2016.

22. Xavier P, Astrup A, Fujioka K, et al. A randomized, controlled trial of 3.0 mg of liraglutide in weight management. N Engl J Med 2015;373:11–22.

23. Gastrointestinal surgery for severe obesity. NIH consens statement online. 1991;9(1):1–20. Available at: https://consensus.nih.gov/1991/1991gisurgeryobesity084html.htm Accessed April 14, 2016.

24. Livingston EH. The incidence of bariatric surgery has plateaued in the U.S. Am J Surg 2010;200(3):378–85. Available at: http://dx.doi.org/10.1016/j.amjsurg.2009.11.007.

25. Wolfe BM, Morton JM. Weighing in on bariatric surgery: procedure use, readmission rates, and mortality. JAMA 2005;294:1960–3.

26. Flum DR, Bell SH, King WC, et al. Perioperative safety in the longitudinal assessment of bariatric surgery. N Engl J Med 2009;361:445–54.

27. Ding S, McKenzie T, Vernon AH, et al. Bariatric Surgery. In: Jameson JL, De Groot JL, editors. Endocrinology: adult and pediatric. 7th edition. Philadelphia: Elsevier/Saunders; 2016. p. 479–90.e4. Chapter 27.

28. Bradley D, Magkos F, Klein S. Effects of Bariatric Surgery on Glucose Homeostasis and Type 2 Diabetes. Gastroenterology 2012;143:897–912. Available at: http://dx.doi.org/10.1053/j.gastro.2012.07.114.

29. Aills L, Blankenship J, Buffington C, et al. ASMBS Allied health nutritional guidelines for the surgical weight loss patient. Surg Obes Relat Dis 2008;4(5 Suppl): S73–108.

30. Harvey JA, Kenny P, Poindexter J, et al. Superior calcium absorption from calcium citrate than calcium carbonate using external forearm counting. J Am Coll Nutr 1990;9(6):583–7.

31. Mechanisk JI, Youdim A, Jones DB, et al. AACE/TOS/ASMBS. clinical practice guidelines for the perioperative nutritional, metabolic, and nonsurgical support of the bariatric surgery patient – 2013 update: cosponsored by American Association of Clinical Endocrinologists, The Obesity Society, and America Society for Metabolic & Bariatric Surgery. Obesity (Silver Spring) 2013;21:s1–27.

32. Stein J, Stier C, Raab H, et al. Review article: the nutritional and pharmacological consequences of obesity surgery. Aliment Pharmacol Ther 2014;40:582–609.

33. Hammond RA, Levine R. The economic impact of obesity in the United States. Diabetes Metab Syndr Obes 2010;3:285–95.

34. O'Grady MJ, Capretta JC. Assessing the economics of obesity and obesity interventions. Washington, DC: Campaign to End Obesity; 2012. Available at: www.obesitycampaign.org http://obesitycampaign.org/documents/StudyAssessingtheEconomicsofObesityandObesityIntervention.pdf. Accessed May 18, 2016.

35. Overweight and obese– fact sheet. Washington, DC: World Health Organization; 2015. Available at: http://www.who.int/mediacentre/factsheets/fs311/en/. Accessed May 18, 2016.

General Pituitary Disorders

Sheila Pinkson, MPAS, BS, PA-C[a,b],*

KEYWORDS

- Pituitary disorder • Hormone • Glands • Neurologic condition

KEY POINTS

- Pituitary disorders can cause hormonal abnormalities that affect the functions of other glands and neurologic conditions.
- Rarely are these disorders life threatening.
- The importance is for early recognition of signs and symptoms of hypersecretion, hyposecretion, and/or mass effects.

PRINCIPLES OF PITUITARY GLAND STRUCTURE AND FUNCTION

The pituitary gland plays a fundamental role in the regulation of many endocrine functions. Often called the master gland, the pituitary hormones influence the secretion of most endocrine glands. Housed in the base of the skull in the area of the sphenoid bone called the sella turcica, the pituitary gland consists of 2 lobes: the anterior and posterior pituitary lobes. Although these 2 lobes are united they are functionally as well as embryologically different. In early development the anterior gland, the adenohypophysis, is derived from the Rathke pouch, a portion of the ectoderm growing superiorly from the roof of the mouth.[1] Most of the pituitary gland is made up of the anterior lobe, which is controlled by hypothalamic hormones that enter the portal veins via the hypophyseal portal system into the anterior lobe.

The posterior lobe, also known as the neurohypophysis, consists of neuronal axons (hypothalamic tract) that originate from the hypothalamus and terminate in the posterior lobe to store hormones. Posterior lobe tissue develops from a protrusion of ectodermal tissue arising from the diencephalon of the developing brain.[1,2] An extension from the hypothalamus, the neural stalk, connects the base hypothalamus to the anterior pituitary gland. **Fig. 1**A shows the basic anatomy of the pituitary gland and **Fig. 1**B shows the embryologic development of the pituitary gland.

The adenohypophysis produces and secretes follicle-stimulating hormone (FSH), luteinizing hormone (LH), adrenocorticotropic hormone (ACTH), melanocyte-stimulating hormone (MSH), thyroid-stimulating hormone (TSH), prolactin (PRL), and growth hormone (GH). The anterior pituitary lobe histologically is categorized into 5

[a] Endocrine, University of Texas Health Science Center at San Antonio, San Antonio, TX, USA;
[b] South Texas Veterans Health Care System, San Antonio, TX, USA
* 7400 Merton Minter Blvd, MC 111, San Antonio, TX 78229.
E-mail address: sheila.pinkson@va.gov

Physician Assist Clin 2 (2017) 107–122
http://dx.doi.org/10.1016/j.cpha.2016.08.009
2405-7991/17/Published by Elsevier Inc.

physicianassistant.theclinics.com

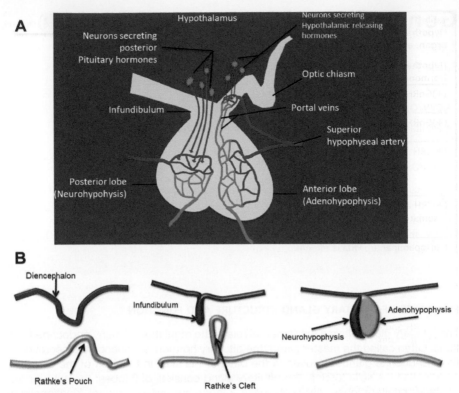

Fig. 1. (*A*) Basic pituitary anatomy. (*B*) Embryologic development of the pituitary gland.

cell types that secrete the corresponding hormone: gonadotrophs (FSH/LH), cortico-trophs (ACTH/MSH), thyrotrophs (TSH), lactotrophs (PRL), and somatotrophs (GH).[3]

Hypothalamic nuclei such as the paraventricular, periventricular, and arcuate nuclei control the anterior pituitary hormone secretion by manufacturing the associated releasing and/or inhibiting hormones. The axons from the hypothalamic nuclei converge into the tuberoinfundibular tract and terminate on the superior hypophyseal artery. The adenohypophysis contains a network of capillaries and connects to the hypothalamus via the hypothalamic-hypophyseal portal system.

Hypothalamic-releasing hormones stimulate the anterior pituitary cell types to discharge hormone into the systemic blood system to reach their target organs. **Table 1** lists the regulating hypothalamic hormones and anterior pituitary hormones classified by cell type, major target organ, and general function. Target organs are generally glandular and, once stimulated by hypothalamic hormones, secrete hormones that can inhibit the release of the tropic in the anterior pituitary and/or inhibit the corresponding hypothalamic-releasing hormone. This process is commonly known as the negative feedback loop. **Fig. 2** shows a simple feedback loop for cortisol.

The neurohypophysis contains axons from the supraoptic and paraventricular hypothalamic nuclei, which form the hypothalamoneurohypophyseal tract. These hypothalamic nuclei produce oxytocin and arginine vasopressin (AVP), also known as antidiuretic hormone (ADH), which is stored for release in the axons housed in the posterior pituitary gland. Neural stimuli cause the release of hormones into circulation. As an example, during lactation, feeding babies activate the hypothalamus to release

Table 1
Hypothalamic hormones and anterior pituitary hormones organized by cell type, target organ, and general function

Hypothalamic Hormone	Anterior Pituitary Hormone	Cell Type	Major Target Organ	Anterior Pituitary Hormone Function
(+)GnRH	FSH	Gonadotrophs	Ovaries/testes	Production of sperm and eggs
(+)GnRH	LH	Gonadotrophs	Ovaries/testes	Production of sex hormones
(+)CRH	ACTH	Corticotrophs	Cortex adrenal gland	Production of glucocorticoids and stress response
(+)TRH and (−) somatostatin	TSH	Thyrotrophs	Thyroid gland	Thyroid hormone release and metabolism
(−)Dopamine	PRL	Lactotrophs	Mammary gland	Female: breast development and milk production. Male: increased sensitivity of LH in testes
(+)GHRH and (−) somatostatin	GH	Somatotrophs	Liver/bone/muscle/ adipose tissue	IGF-1 secretion and body growth, increased metabolic rate

Minus symbols indicate inhibition; plus symbols indicate stimulation.
Abbreviations: CRH, corticotropin-releasing hormone; GHRH, growth hormone–releasing hormone; GnRH, gonadotropin-releasing hormone; IGF-1, insulinlike growth factor-1; TRH, thyrotropin-releasing hormone.

oxytocin, stimulating mammary glands to expel milk. Other neural stimuli, such as a mother reminiscing about her baby, can activate this response to let down her milk. During dehydration the hypothalamus senses hyperosmolality in the blood and sends stimuli to the supraoptic and paraventricular nuclei to release AVP in the blood stream. AVP decreases serum osmolality and increases free water absorption in the kidney via the distal convoluted tubule and collecting ducts. This water retention increases blood pressure and regulates water balance sensed by the hypothalamus and other receptors to stop AVP release. **Table 2** lists the hormones stored in the posterior pituitary gland, major target organs, and general function.

DISORDERS OF PITUITARY HORMONE AXIS

Endocrine pituitary disorders can manifest from either a hyperfunctioning or hypofunctioning gland from multiple causes. Pituitary gland disorders can affect the biochemical processes needed to maintain the body's metabolism. In addition, neurologic disorders can develop from pituitary disorders because of the anatomic proximity of pituitary tumors to other nerve structures (ie, cranial nerves). This article reviews general pituitary disorders and conditions.

Pituitary Adenomas: Classification

The incidence of pituitary adenomas is 17% to 20% within the general population.[4,5] Commonly, pituitary adenomas are benign monoclonal adenomas derived from cells

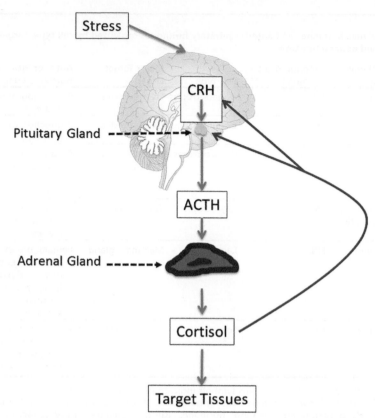

Fig. 2. Simple feedback loop for cortisol secretion through the hypothalamic-pituitary-adrenal axis.

located in the anterior pituitary gland. Pituitary neoplasms can be classified as functioning or nonfunctioning lesions. One of the 5 cell types (lactotrophs, somatotrophs, gonadotrophs, corticotrophs, and less commonly thyrotrophs) in the adenohypophysis determines the type of functioning adenoma, which clinically presents with signs and symptoms of hormone excess. Pituitary adenomas can also be classified by size,

Table 2			
Hypothalamic secreting neurons, hormones stored in the posterior pituitary gland, target organ, and hormone function			
Hypothalamic Neurons	Neurohypophysial Hormone	Target Organ	Hormone Function
Supraoptic nucleus	Oxytocin	Uterus, mammary glands	Women: uterine contractions and milk let-down during lactation
Paraventricular nucleus	Vasopressin (ADH)	Kidneys	Water reabsorption: increased water permeability at the distal convoluted tubules and collecting ducts

whereby lesions less than 10 mm in diameter are defined as microadenomas and those greater than 10 mm are considered macroadenomas. **Fig. 3** shows MRI sella views for a normal pituitary and a macroadenoma. In addition, pituitary axis disorders can occur despite the adenoma size.

Mass effects emerge when the macroadenoma encroaches beyond the sella. These mass effects include headaches, visual field deficits, partial/panhypopituitarism, seizures, and cranial nerve defects. Classically, pituitary adenomas are associated with bitemporal hemianopsia when the adenoma compresses the optic chiasm, causing visual field loss in the temporal fields bilaterally but maintaining eyesight in the nasal fields. However, incomplete bitemporal defects are more commonly seen. These visual deficits depend on tumor size, location, and proximity to the optic chiasm. **Fig. 4** compares normal vision with temporal deficits from compression of the optic chiasm. Early recognition in patients with visual defects, gonadal dysfunction, and headaches by clinicians should raise a red flag for urgent MRI in addition to referral to endocrinology and neurosurgery.[6]

Secretory Tumors/Functioning Adenomas

Prolactinoma

Prolactin-secreting adenomas arise from lactotrophic cells in the anterior pituitary gland. Prolactinomas are the most common pituitary tumors and comprise 40% of all pituitary tumors.[7] In general, prolactinomas are slow-growing microadenomas and are more prevalent in women. Giant prolactinomas, those larger than 4 cm, are infrequent, making up 2% to 3% of all prolactin tumors, and are more common in men.[8]

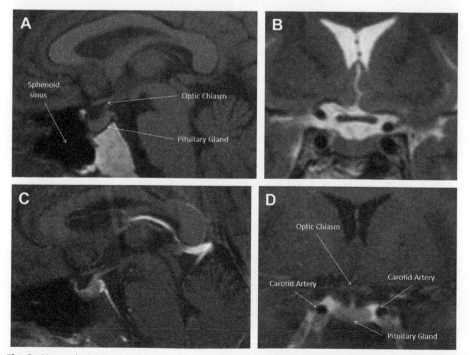

Fig. 3. Normal pituitary sella in a 35-year-old male patient. (*A*) T1 sagittal; (*B*) T2 coronal; (*C*) postgadolinium T1 sagittal, fat saturated; (*D*) postgadolinium T1 coronal, fat saturated.

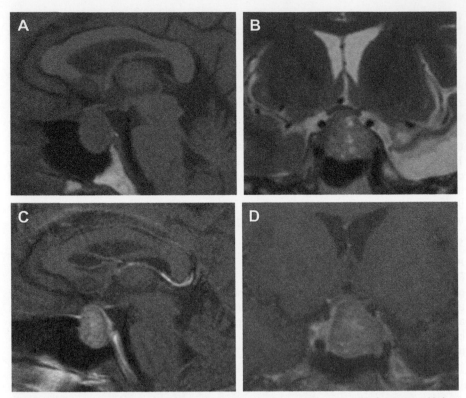

Fig. 4. Pituitary macroadenoma found in 36-year old man with history of left temporal lobectomy. (*A*) T1 sagittal, (*B*) T2-weighted coronal, (*C*) postgadolinium T1 sagittal, (*D*) postgadolinium T1 coronal. Pituitary tumor measured 1.5 × 1.6 × 1.6 cm (AP × CC × TR). Note the mass abutting the optic chiasm. AP, anteroposterior; CC, craniocaudel; TR, transverse.

The main function of prolactin is to establish mammary gland tissue during pregnancy and milk production. Increased prolactin levels cause hypogonadism by blocking the pulsatile secretion of gonadotropin-releasing hormone (GnRH) as well as directly inhibiting FSH. Estrogen stimulates prolactin excretion. Inhibitory control arises from increases in dopamine levels that originate from tuberoinfundibular-pituitary neurons overruling hypothalamic stimulation.[8] Signs and symptoms of increased prolactin levels in women are irregular menses/amenorrhea, infertility, decreased libido, and galactorrhea. In men, hyperprolactinemia manifests as decreased sperm count, decreased libido, and sometimes gynecomastia (milk production is very rare). Chronic prolactin level increase can cause decreased bone mineral density because of prolonged hypogonadism. In general, transient hyperprolactinemia is most often seen in pregnancy and breastfeeding, which is physiologic and resolves once completed. Pathologic hyperprolactinemia needs further treatment to impede the effects of increased prolactin level, prevent tumor enlargement, and reduce mass effects. **Table 3** lists the signs and symptoms of hyperprolactinemia.

A serum prolactin level should be drawn if hyperprolactinemia is suspected. Prolactin levels are usually proportional to tumor size. Microprolactinomas have serum prolactin levels from 100 to 200 ng/mL. Serum prolactin levels in macroprolactinomas tend to be

Table 3 Sign/symptoms of hyperprolactinemia	
Male	**Female**
• Testosterone deficiency	• Estrogen insufficiency
○ Decreased libido	○ Amenorrhea/oligomenorrhea
○ Erectile dysfunction	○ Irregular menses
○ Decreased sperm quality/motility	○ Infertility
○ Infertility	• Galactorrhea
• Galactorrhea (very rare)	• Chronic increase
• Chronic increase	○ Osteopenia/osteoporosis
○ Osteopenia/osteoporosis	

greater than or equal to 200 ng/mL.[7] Note that stalk compression from nonfunctioning pituitary tumors can cause modest increase in prolactin level. Therefore, only mildly increased (30–70s ng/mL) prolactin levels with macroadenoma should raise the suspicion of nonfunctional adenoma rather than prolactin-producing adenoma.

A complete history and physical examination is imperative to rule out nonpituitary causes of prolactinemia. In women it is important to exclude pregnancy first. Nipple/chest stimulation may turn on afferent pathways to the hypothalamus, causing increased prolactin levels. In addition, TSH level should be evaluated because chronic hypothyroidism has been known to increase serum prolactin levels by thyrotropin-releasing hormone (TRH) stimulation. Renal insufficiency and hepatic failure are other causes of hyperprolactinemia because of decreased clearance. A thorough review of the patient's medication list should be completed to determine whether medications or supplements are disrupting dopamine secretion and causing a drug-induced hyperprolactinemia (eg, neuroleptics, atypical antipsychotics, metoclopramide, verapamil, methyldopa, estrogen).[7,9] During the physical examination, it is important to evaluate extraocular movements (ophthalmoplegia), visual fields by confrontation (visual field defects), presence of galactorrhea (in premenopausal women), signs of hypothyroidism, and hypogonadism. If the work-up suggests a prolactinoma, then a pituitary MRI with and without contrast should be ordered.

Most patients respond to therapy within weeks of initiation, as shown by symptoms and prolactin levels. The main therapeutic goal for treatment of prolactinomas is to reduce prolactin to normal levels and decrease the tumor's size, especially in macroprolactinomas. Signs and symptoms of tumor mass effects and decreased gonadal function will be restored when prolactin levels improve. Most patients have more than a 25% decrease in the size of the adenoma. Usually, dopamine agonists are the treatment of choice. Having better efficacy in decreasing serum prolactin level and decreasing tumor size, cabergoline is preferred to other dopamine agonists.[9] Cabergoline is taken less frequently (usually twice a week) compared with other agents (daily), which is another advantage. Resistant prolactinomas, defined as those unresponsive to dopamine agonists, may need referral to surgery if suboptimal response to maximum dopamine agonists is noted.

Growth hormone–secreting tumors (gigantism/acromegaly)
Acromegaly is a protracted disorder caused by excessive secretion of GH in adults. Gigantism is the same disorder except the hypersecretion occurs in children/adolescents whose epiphyseal plates have not yet matured into the epiphyseal line. The major cause of acromegaly is hypersecreting somatotroph cells from a pituitary adenoma.[10] GH circulates in the blood and stimulates the liver to produce insulinlike

growth factor-1 (IGF-1).[11] The IGF-1 facilitates tissue and bone proliferation, leading to overgrowth and metabolic dysfunction. In normal patients, IGF-1 aids in regulating GH secretion along with somatostatin secreted by the hypothalamus. Normally GH secretion is inhibited by somatostatin and IGF-1. Acromegaly/gigantism arises from autonomous GH production that is unresponsive to suppression from somatostatin or IGF-1. The insidious growth of these GH pituitary adenomas occurs over several years and they are generally found as macroadenomas that compress surrounding brain tissue, causing mass effects and nerve damage.

The clinical manifestations of acromegaly typically include coarse facial features, prognathism, and enlarged spade hands and feet. Bone growth and tissue swelling result in prominent supraorbital ridges, and enlarged nose, lips, and macroglossia leading to sleep apnea. In addition, a deep husky voice change indicates larynx enlargement. Headaches are common and most likely caused by the enlargement of the pituitary tumor. Visual field defects may be present because of the same disorders. Other organs expand as well, such as the heart, thyroid, pancreas, and kidneys. Cardiomegaly and cardiomyopathy often develop. Other tumor compression nerve disorders may occur. Skin tags and colon polyps can develop, and periodic monitoring with colonoscopy is indicated. Decreases in gonadotropin level can occur, leading to abnormal menstruation and decreased libido. Chronic increases of GH levels are associated with insulin resistance and patients are at increased risk of developing diabetes mellitus.[12,13]

Patients with signs or symptoms of acromegaly should first be evaluated with serum IGF-1. Serum IGF-1 level is the initial key laboratory value to obtain in acromegaly, because IGF-1 has a longer serum half-life and levels remain fairly stable compared with serum GH levels, which has a shorter half-life, is pulsatile, and the level peaks overnight, which makes it a poor choice for a screening test. IGF-1 levels correlate well with GH activity. If serum IGF-1 level is increased, a GH suppression test should be performed with an oral glucose loading test. After a 75-g oral glucose load is ingested, the diagnosis is confirmed if GH level does not suppress to less than 1 μg/mL. An MRI scan of the pituitary sella should be performed, if not contraindicated, to assess size, location, and extent of parasellar tumor involvement.[10] Patients showing symptoms of acromegaly should also be evaluated for the possible comorbidities of sleep apnea, diabetes mellitus, hypertension, and osteoarthritis.

Acromegaly-associated morbidity and mortality are increased because of end-organ effects of increased IGF-1 levels, including tumor mass consequences and associated comorbidities. The primary treatment strategy is to normalize GH and IGF-1 levels, reduce symptoms, and control tumor mass.[10,11] If the tumor is judged to be resectable, transsphenoidal resection is the most common treatment modality. Experienced surgeons can improve clinical outcomes for more than 40% of macroadenomas and more than 85% of microadenomas.[10] Hypopituitarism may be caused by surgery or by tumor compression. Other complications of surgery are nasal congestion, changes in taste olfactory sensation, cerebrospinal fluid leak, infection, diabetes insipidus (transient/permanent), and death.[13] Patients with large tumors that are difficult to resect may need further surgery/medical therapy. Persistent disease despite surgery may require somatostatin receptor ligands (ie, octreotide) and/or GH receptor antagonists. In addition, radiotherapy should be considered in those patients who are unable to tolerate medical therapy or where medicines are unavailable.

Cushing disease
ACTH-producing tumors cause Cushing disease. An excess of cortisol is produced by the overstimulation of the adrenal cortex by ACTH. Cushing disease should not to be

confused with Cushing syndrome, which refers to general excess of serum cortisol regardless of the cause (endogenous or exogenous sources of glucocorticoids). **Box 1** describes the clinical features of Cushing syndrome.[14] Cushing disease is considered rare and the incidence is estimated to be 1.2 to 2.4 cases per million inhabitants per year.[14] These pituitary tumors are corticotropin-producing adenomas and are usually benign. Rarely, Cushing disease is associated with multiple endocrine neoplasia type 1 (MEN1), caused by a genetic mutation of the menin gene in an autosomal dominant pattern and associated with parathyroid tumors, pancreatic endocrine tumors, and pituitary adenomas.[14] Uncommon in children, Cushing disease most commonly affects adults between 20 and 40 years of age, with most being women of childbearing age.[14,15]

The clinical characteristics of Cushing disease show more typical features of chronic cortisol excess compared with an ectopic ACTH syndrome. Excess cortisol features such as purple striae, paper-thin skin, easy bruising, and proximal muscle

---

Box 1
Sign/symptoms of Cushing syndrome

- Obesity
  - Dorsal and supraclavicular fat pads (so-called buffalo hump)
  - Rounded face (so-called moon facies)
  - Central obesity

- Protein wasting
  - Muscle wasting (lower extremity atrophy)
  - Proximal muscle weakness
  - Cutaneous atrophy
    - Purple striae (abdomen, breasts, axilla, hips)
    - Easy bruising
    - Poor wound healing

- Bone disturbances
  - Bone pain or tenderness
  - Osteopenia/osteoporosis
  - Hypocalcemia

- Hypertension

- Impaired immunity

- Gonadal dysfunction
  - Hyperandrogenism
  - Facial hirsutism
  - Female balding
  - Menstrual disturbances
    - Oligomenorrhea/amenorrhea
  - Impotence
  - Acne

- Diabetes mellitus
  - Polydipsia
  - Polyuria
  - Blurry vision
  - Fatigue

- Psychological disturbances
  - Depression
  - Anxiety
  - Mood swings/irritability

weakness develop over a longer period of time (1–2 years) are more common with Cushing disease compared with ectopic presentations.[16] Other common manifestations include rounded facial features, described as moon facies, weight gain, truncal obesity, supraclavicular and dorsocervical fat pads creating the classic so-called buffalo hump, and muscular atrophy.[15] Pituitary mass effects can also develop, causing visual field defects, headaches, and nerve palsy. Clinically patients often develop uncontrolled diabetes mellitus, hypertension, and osteoporosis.

Timely diagnosis and intervention are important, because untreated Cushing disease increases morbidity and mortality. Because Cushing syndrome is most commonly iatrogenic, it is important to review the patient's medical record and history to rule out exogenous glucocorticoid exposure. Patients with features of Cushing syndrome should be biochemically evaluated. The Endocrine Society recommends one of the following: urine free cortisol level (at minimum 2 measurements), late night salivary cortisol level (at minimum 2 measurements), an overnight 1-mg dexamethasone suppression test, or a 48-hour 2-mg dexamethasone suppression test. If any abnormal test suggests hypercortisolism, then the next step is to determine whether the hypercortisolemia is ACTH dependent (driven by increased ACTH level leading to overproduction of cortisol from adrenal cortex) versus ACTH independent (autonomous hyperfunctioning adrenal cortex/adenoma suppressing hypothalamus/pituitary, suppressed ACTH). Random serum ACTH testing (without dexamethasone administration) showing high to high normal levels suggests the ACTH-dependent form, and low to low normal levels suggest the ACTH-independent form. Cushing disease is ACTH dependent. An MRI sella can confirm Cushing disease if the adenoma is greater than 6 mm with concordant laboratory values with ACTH-dependent hypercortisolemia.[14] If MRI is nonconfirmatory for an adenoma despite positive biochemical results, then a bilateral intrapetrosal sinus sampling can be conducted to confirm ACTH-dependent hypercortisolism.

First-line treatment of Cushing disease is transsphenoidal surgery. Remission rates range from 50% to 70%.[14] Patients with recurrent or persistent hypercortisolism may need additional treatment, such as surgery, radiotherapy, and/or medical therapy. Some examples of medication for second-line treatment include steroidogenesis inhibitors such as ketoconazole. Ketoconazole is primarily used as an antifungal agent and should be used with caution because it inhibits cytochrome P450 enzymes. In addition, glucocorticoid receptor antagonists like mifepristone may be used. A new option is pasireotide, a somatostatin analogue that has a high affinity to somatostatin receptor subtype 5 and is also found in corticotroph adenomas and works to inhibit corticotropin secretion. Bilateral adrenalectomy is considered in patients who have failed pituitary surgery or with severe hypercortisolism. Nelson syndrome, characterized by hyperpigmentation, enlargement of the ACTH-secreting pituitary adenoma, and increased ACTH levels, may develop after total adrenalectomy because of lack of pituitary inhibition from cortisol. The tumor's aggressiveness and advancing size contribute to increased morbidity and mortality. Cushing disease is not only challenging to diagnose but also difficult to manage.

Thyrotropin pituitary adenomas

Thyrotropin pituitary adenomas are very rare. Approximately 2% of pituitary tumors are thyrotropin-secreting adenomas, as reported in surgical series.[17] There have been more than 450 thyrotropin-secreting tumor cases reported in the medical literature since first being described in 1960. Most patients with these tumors are in their fifth or sixth decade of life.

Patient's with thyrotropin-secreting adenomas present with typical findings of mild hyperthyroidism, which include increased thyroid hormone levels, weight loss, palpitations, tremors, and heat intolerance. In addition, most of the thyrotrophic tumors are invasive macroadenomas causing mass effect symptoms. Goiter is present because of chronic TSH stimulation. Hypopituitarism develops in some patients.

Biochemically, TSH level is increased or normal in the presence of increased free T4. MRI sella is the imaging study of choice to detect a pituitary adenoma. Given the rarity of this disorder, it is prudent to refer to an endocrinologist who can distinguish between a thyrotropin-secreting adenoma versus resistance to thyroid hormone, because both disorders present with increased free thyroid levels in the presence of a normal or increased TSH level.[18]

As with many pituitary tumors, surgery is first-line therapy, especially for macroadenomas, in order to quell signs and symptoms and relieve mass effects. Studies have shown that somatostatin analogues can not only inhibit GH release but also block thyrotropin response to TRH.[19] However, somatostatin analogues are not regarded as first-line therapy but are used in combination therapeutic regimens. Radiation therapy is another option that is often used for persistent/recurrent disease.

Nonsecretory Tumors/Nonfunctioning Pituitary Adenomas

Nonfunctioning pituitary adenomas are tumors that do not cause an oversecretion of pituitary hormones. Almost all of these adenomas are derived from gonadotrophic cells, and a smaller group is made up of the other trophic cell lines. Again, these adenomas do not cause excessive hormone levels.[20]

Many of these nonsecretory tumors are found incidentally on computed tomography (CT) or MRI studies. Larger tumors manifest the typical mass effect signs and symptoms depending on compromised areas. Patients with macroadenomas and even larger microincidentalomas (6–9 mm) should undergo further hormone evaluation.[17] Macroadenomas are more associated with hypopituitarism. In addition, a baseline visual field examination is indicated for macroadenomas. Nonfunctioning microadenomas should have a repeat MRI scan in 1 year and then yearly for 3 years, then tapered to lesser frequency if the size is stable. In nonfunctioning macroadenomas, if a patient has abnormal visual field testing or hypopituitarism is present, surgery is recommended.[6] In the absence of these signs and symptoms, repeating MRI and biochemical pituitary evaluation in 6 months is recommended. Monitored patients developing pituitary growth on imaging or visual field deficit should be referred to surgery. **Fig. 5** presents the Endocrine Society flow diagram for pituitary incidentalomas.

Nonpituitary Sella Masses

Rathke cleft cyst
Rathke cleft cyst is a benign sella or suprasellar mass derived from vestiges of the Rathke pouch. It is made up of mucinous material that consists of cholesterol and protein that appears hyperintense on T1 MRI. In general, Rathke cleft cysts are small and asymptomatic and do not require surgical intervention. However, Rathke cleft cysts that are large enough may cause pressure on adjoining structures, causing headaches, visual field deficits, and pituitary hormone disturbances.

These cysts are among the most common incidentally found sellar lesions. Commonly, imaging on CT or MRI shows an ovoid or dumbbell-shaped lesion in the pars intermedia, the area between the posterior and anterior pituitary lobes. **Fig. 6** shows a Rathke cleft cyst on MRI. On MRI there are typical cystic findings with little cell wall enhancement.[21] For symptomatic patients, providers should complete a biochemical work-up for hypopituitarism.

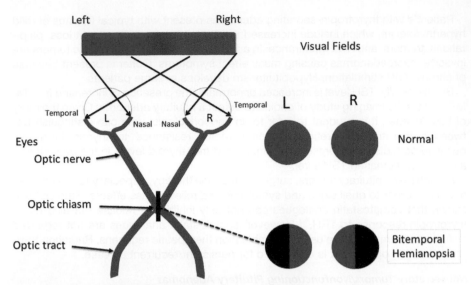

Fig. 5. Normal visual fields versus bitemporal hemianopsia.

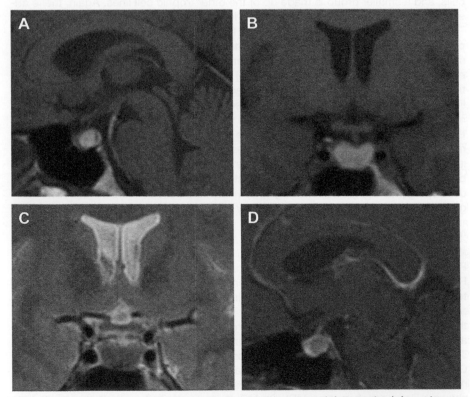

Fig. 6. Rathke cleft cyst on MRI sella in a 42-year-old woman. (*A*) T1 sagittal, hyperintense cyst; (*B*) T1 noncontrast coronal, hyperintense; (*C*) T2 coronal, hypointense lesion; (*D*) post-gadolinium T1 sagittal nonenhancing (posterior sella).

Treatment of symptomatic Rathke cleft cysts is draining the lesion and removing the capsule. The goal of therapy is to relieve visual field disturbances and preserve the pituitary hormone axis.

Craniopharyngiomas

Another rare tumor derived from malformation of embryonic tissue, possibly from the Rathke pouch, is a craniopharyngioma. This tumor occurs in the sellar or parasellar area of the brain. Most common is suprasellar lesions, whereas intrasellar lesions are the least common.[22]

Depending on the location of the lesion, craniopharyngiomas can present with signs/symptoms of mass effect. The diagnosis is sometimes delayed because of nonspecific conditions such as headache and nausea. In adults, visual field disturbances and hormone deficiencies are more evident than in children. Around 40% to 80% of patients with craniopharyngiomas have at least 1 hormone insufficiency.[22]

The treatment goal is to resect the tumor while preserving pituitary function and other neurologic structures. Neurosurgery is a good option for tumors within the sella. Complicated tumors involving the hypothalamus are more challenging and may need surgery and irradiation. Depending on the tumor involvement, treatment may cause additional hormone deficiencies, and cranial nerve deficits. Hypothalamic obesity, daytime sleepiness, and behavioral changes can be evident with hypothalamus involvement.[22]

Empty Sella Syndrome

Empty sella syndrome is a condition in which the cerebrospinal fluid fills the sella turcica and compresses the pituitary gland against the bone. Primary empty sella results from anatomic conditions in which the cerebrospinal fluid enters through a sellar diaphragm. Secondary empty sella occurs through pituitary surgery/irradiation or pituitary injury.[23]

Evaluation with MRI shows either an empty or partially empty sella. The pituitary gland is commonly not affected. However, there are rare incidents in which there is pituitary dysfunction or abnormal function. Patients who show any clinical manifestation of hormonal abnormalities should undergo a biochemical work-up.

Central Diabetes Insipidus

Central diabetes insipidus (CDI) is the abnormal reduction of the level of ADH, also known as arginine vasopressin (AVP). AVP deficiency causes polyuria, polydipsia, and nocturia. Idiopathic diabetes insipidus is the most common cause of CDI. Other causes are pituitary or parasellar tumors, neurosurgery, and brain trauma. Postsurgical diabetes insipidus is sometimes transient. There are also hereditary cases of familial diabetes insipidus.

CDI can involve complete or partial obliteration of AVP secretion. Patients consume excessive liquids daily, from 3 to 30 L. Urine is very dilute because AVP is not present or is insufficient to concentrate urine and increase serum osmolality. Urine specific gravity is low (<1.005), and serum sodium levels are high or high normal. To assist in diagnosis, a water deprivation test is done under close supervision. Persistent CDI may cause neurologic symptoms, hypovolemia, and dehydration if left untreated.

Replacement with a synthetic vasopressin, desmopressin, is the treatment of CDI. Preparations are commonly intranasal solutions but can be given by oral, subcutaneous, or parenteral administration. The goal is to improve patients' signs and symptoms, achieve normal serum sodium levels and improved fluid retention, and avoid hyponatremia.

Pituitary Apoplexy

A rare endocrine emergency, pituitary apoplexy is an acute hemorrhage or infarction of the pituitary gland. Pituitary apoplexy is usually associated with pituitary adenomas and occurs in 0.6% to 10% of surgically treated pituitary adenomas.[24] However, this condition can also occur in hypophysitis, craniopharyngioma, and Rathke cleft cyst. Many cases occur in the fifth or sixth decade with a male preponderance.

Symptoms of pituitary apoplexy occur within hours to a few days. Classically, patients complain of headache, visual defects, diplopia, ptosis, and ophthalmoplegia. Interruption of the pituitary gland blood supply causes pituitary hormone deficiency in 80% of patients. In particular, 70% of patients with pituitary apoplexy develop ACTH deficiency, 50% TSH deficiency, and 75% gonadotropin deficiency in reviewed cases.[24] Patients with hypocortisolism have acquired hyponatremia. In addition, hemorrhage in the pituitary gland can cause rapid mass effect symptoms.

CT imaging in the acute setting can show recent hemorrhage within the first 3 hours and shows hyperdensity. However, MRI is more sensitive in identifying pituitary tumor and hemorrhage compared with CT. MRI can be used to follow the lesion months and years after apoplexy.[24]

Pituitary apoplexy needs immediate medical management, to include maintenance of hemodynamic stability, fluid and electrolyte balance, and glucocorticoid replacement. Treatment can be surgical or conservative management depending on the assessments and evaluation of the multidisciplinary team. Long-term follow-up is needed to monitor recurrence and hormonal function.

Sheehan Syndrome

Similar to apoplexy, Sheehan syndrome is an ischemic pituitary event that occurs after delivery. This syndrome is caused by pituitary ischemia from excessive postpartum hemorrhage. The combination of increased pituitary volume during pregnancy, postpartum hypotension, and reduced blood flow in the pituitary gland can trigger pituitary necrosis.

In Sheehan syndrome, pituitary hormone production is reduced and the reduction depends on the amount of pituitary necrosis or damage. There should be a high suspicion in a postpartum woman with hypotension and hypoglycemia. Other presentations include inability to lactate, and amenorrhea. In addition, patients may experience extreme fatigue, dizziness, muscle weakness, hyponatremia, and cold intolerance from other anterior pituitary hormone deficiencies. However, diabetes insipidus and hypernatremia can also be present.

CT and MRI can be useful. During an acute phase, CT may show an enlarged pituitary gland. Serial imaging weeks after insult may show an atrophic gland or empty sella.

Treatment of Sheehan syndrome entails hormone replacement depending on the type of deficiency. Secondary adrenal insufficiency should be assessed before thyroid hormone replacement. Adrenal crisis may occur if an undiagnosed secondary adrenal insufficiency is first replaced with thyroid hormone.

SUMMARY

Pituitary disorders can cause hormonal abnormalities that affect the functions of other glands and neurologic conditions. Rarely are these disorders life threatening. However, there are multiple and sometimes subtle manifestations of these pituitary disorders that can provide a significant challenge in the diagnoses and management of many pituitary conditions. The importance is for early recognition of signs and symptoms of hypersecretion, hyposecretion, and/or mass effects. A multidisciplinary approach should be coordinated with an endocrinologist and other specialties to provide management and follow-up for the best treatment practices.

REFERENCES

1. Childs GV. Pituitary gland (cell types, mediators, development) A2-Squire. In: Larry R, editor. Encyclopedia of neuroscience. Oxford (United Kingdom): Academic Press; 2009. p. 719–26.
2. Davis SW, Ellsworth BS, Peréz Millan MI, et al. Pituitary gland development and disease: from stem cell to hormone production. Curr Top Dev Biol 2013;106:1–47.
3. Ooi GT, Tawadros N, Escalona RM. Pituitary cell lines and their endocrine applications. Mol Cell Endocrinol 2004;228:1–21.
4. Theodros D, Patel M, Ruzevick J, et al. Pituitary adenomas: historical perspective, surgical management and future directions. CNS Oncol 2015;4:411–29.
5. Scangas GA, Laws ER Jr. Pituitary incidentalomas. Pituitary 2014;17:486–91.
6. Freda PU, Beckers AM, Katznelson L, et al. Pituitary incidentaloma: an Endocrine Society clinical practice guideline. J Clin Endocrinol Metab 2011;96:894–904.
7. Wong A, Eloy JA, Couldwell WT, et al. Update on prolactinomas. Part 1: clinical manifestations and diagnostic challenges. J Clin Neurosci 2015;22:1562–7.
8. Glezer A, Bronstein MD. Prolactinomas. Endocrinol Metab Clin North Am 2015; 44:71–8.
9. Melmed S, Casanueva FF, Hoffman AR, et al. Diagnosis and treatment of hyperprolactinemia: an Endocrine Society clinical practice guideline. J Clin Endocrinol Metab 2011;96:273–88.
10. Katznelson L, Laws ER Jr, Melmed S, et al. Acromegaly: an endocrine society clinical practice guideline. J Clin Endocrinol Metab 2014;99:3933–51.
11. Giustina A, Chanson P, Bronstein MD, et al. A consensus on criteria for cure of acromegaly. J Clin Endocrinol Metab 2010;95:3141–8.
12. Ayuk J, Sheppard MC. Growth hormone and its disorders. Postgrad Med J 2006; 82:24–30.
13. Capatina C, Wass JAH. 60 Years of neuroendocrinology: acromegaly. J Endocrinol 2015;226:T141–60.
14. Castinetti F, Morange I, Conte-Devolx B, et al. Cushing's disease. Orphanet J Rare Dis 2012;7:1–9.
15. De Martin M, Giraldi FP, Cavagnini F. Cushing's disease. Pituitary 2006;9:279–87.
16. Daniel E, Newell-Price JD. Diagnosis of Cushing's disease. Pituitary 2015;18: 206–10.
17. Orija IB, Weil RJ, Hamrahian AH. Pituitary incidentaloma. Best Pract Res Clin Endocrinol Metab 2012;26:47–68.
18. Beck-Peccoz P, Persani L, Mannavola D, et al. Pituitary tumours: TSH-secreting adenomas. Best Pract Res Clin Endocrinol Metab 2009;23:597–606.
19. Amlashi FG, Tritos NA. Thyrotropin-secreting pituitary adenomas: epidemiology, diagnosis, and management. Endocrine 2016;52:427–40.
20. Molitch ME. Pituitary incidentalomas. Best Pract Res Clin Endocrinol Metab 2009; 23:667–75.
21. Trifanescu R, Ansorge O, Wass JA, et al. Rathke's cleft cysts. Clin Endocrinol 2012;76:151–60.
22. Muller HL. Craniopharyngioma. Endocr Rev 2014;35:513–43.

23. Huguet I, Clayton R. Pituitary-hypothalamic tumor syndromes: adults. In: De Groot LJ, Beck-Peccoz P, Chrousos G, et al, editors. Endotext. South Dartmouth (MA): MDText.com, Inc; 2000. Available at: www.endotext.org.
24. Glezer A, Bronstein MD. Pituitary apoplexy: pathophysiology, diagnosis and management. Arch Endocrinol Metab 2015;59:259–64.

Adrenal Disorders
Beyond the "Flight or Fight" Response

Kristen A. Scheckel, PA-C

KEYWORDS

- Congenital adrenal hyperplasia • Adrenal insufficiency • Cushing syndrome
- Primary aldosteronism/Conn syndrome • Pheochromocytoma

KEY POINTS

- The diagnosis of adrenal disorders is based on clinical findings, biochemical and hormonal laboratory values, and imaging results, often with multiple confounding factors making the diagnosis challenging.
- Replacement of deficient hormones in congenital adrenal hyperplasia and adrenal insufficiency is crucial for reducing morbidity and mortality associated with these conditions.
- In cortisol-deficient states, a top priority is patient education regarding stress dosing of glucocorticoid therapy during illness, surgery, or trauma and management of adrenal crisis. These patients should carry a medical alert card or necklace/bracelet at all times denoting their diagnosis, medications, and emergency plan.
- In conditions involving hormone excess, such as Cushing syndrome, primary aldosteronism, and pheochromocytoma, the primary goal is to determine the source/location of hormone excess and then proceed with either surgical resection or medication intervention to normalize excessive hormone levels.

ADRENAL GLAND ANATOMY

The adrenal glands are paired organs located in the retroperitoneum, superior to the upper poles of the kidneys.[1] Each adrenal gland contains an outer cortex and an inner medulla. The cortex is comprised of three zones that synthesize steroid hormones. The outer zona glomerulosa produces mineralocorticoids, mainly aldosterone. The central zona fasciculata produces glucocorticoids, primarily cortisol. The inner zona reticularis secretes androgens, mainly dehydroepiandrostenedione (DHEA), DHEA sulfate (DHES-S), and testosterone.[2,3] The medulla is the site of catecholamine production (**Figs. 1 and 2**).[3]

DISORDERS OF ADRENAL STEROIDOGENESIS
Background

All adrenal steroid hormones are made from cholesterol through multiple steps outlined in **Fig. 3**.[4] Disorders of adrenal steroidogenesis can involve either overproduction or underproduction of steroids depending on the specific enzyme defect. The most

The author has nothing to disclose.
3865 E. Cherry Creek North Drive, Suite 322, Denver, CO 80209, USA
E-mail address: kascheckel@gmail.com

Physician Assist Clin 2 (2017) 123–139
http://dx.doi.org/10.1016/j.cpha.2016.08.010   **physicianassistant.theclinics.com**

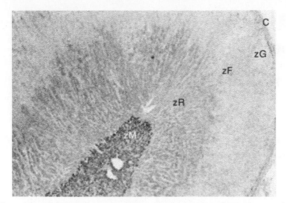

Fig. 1. Cross-sectional image of a human adrenal gland. C, adrenal capsule; zF, zona fascic-ulate; zG, zona glomerulosa; zM, adrenal medulla; zR, zona reticularis. (*From* Vrezas I, Wil-lenberg HS, Bornstein SR. Adrenal cortex, anatomy. In: Martini L, editor. Encyclopedia of endocrine diseases, vol. I. 1st edition. Academic Press; 2004. p. 50; with permission.)

common enzyme defects affect cortisol production and are collectively referred to as congenital adrenal hyperplasia (CAH).[5] Reduced cortisol production results in lack of negative feedback to the hypothalamus and pituitary, which results in chronic eleva-tion of corticotropin-releasing hormone (CRH) and adrenocorticotropic hormone

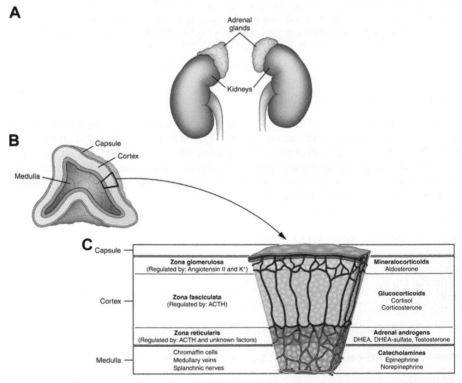

Fig. 2. (*A–C*) Structure and function of the layers of the adrenal gland. ACTH, adrenocorti-cotropic hormone. (*From* Norman AW, Henry HL. Adrenal corticoids. [Chapter 10]. In: Hor-mones. 3rd edition. Academic Press; 2015. p. 224.)

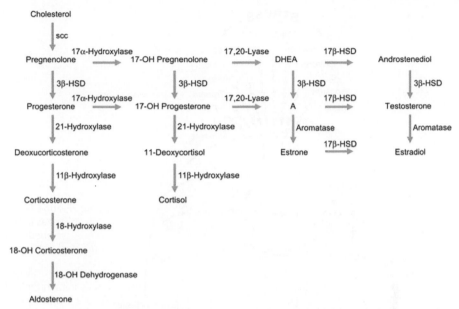

Fig. 3. Biochemical pathways of adrenal steroid synthesis. (*Data from* Nicolaides NC, Charmandari E, Chrousos GP. Adrenal steroid hormone secretion: physiologic and endocrine aspects. In: Reference module in biomedical research. 3rd edition. 2014. p. 3.)

(ACTH), leading to overstimulation of the adrenal cortex by ACTH and eventual adrenal hyperplasia (**Fig. 4**).[5]

Classic CAH is defined by significantly reduced enzyme activity with impaired cortisol production manifesting at birth. Nonclassic forms of CAH result from less severe enzyme defects and symptoms are milder, typically without genital ambiguity. Nonclassic CAH is more prevalent than classic CAH.[1,6] Approximately 90% to 95% of cases of CAH are caused by 21-hydroxylase enzyme deficiency. All forms of CAH are transmitted in an autosomal-recessive pattern.[5]

Screening for CAH at birth is currently performed in all 50 states in the United States.[5] Every newborn with ambiguous genitalia or persistently undescended testes should be karyotyped for chromosomal sex and evaluated for classic 21-hydroxylase deficiency.[1]

Clinical Features

In 21-hydroxylase deficiency, upstream steroid precursors (17-hydroxyprogesterone [17-OHP], progesterone, 17-hydroxypregnenolone, and pregnenolone) accumulate and are diverted to form androgens.[5] Excess adrenal androgen production results in genital ambiguity and virilization in females.[1] Males with CAH do not exhibit genital ambiguity at birth.[5]

Severe mutations in the 21-hydroxylase enzyme also result in impaired aldosterone synthesis, called classic salt wasting 21-hydroxylase deficiency. Approximately 75% of patients with classic CAH have the salt wasting form with potentially fatal hypovolemia, hypoglycemia, and shock.[6]

Diagnosis

In classic CAH, baseline serum cortisol levels are in the low range and serum 17-OHP and adrenal androgens are significantly elevated, often 100-times higher than the

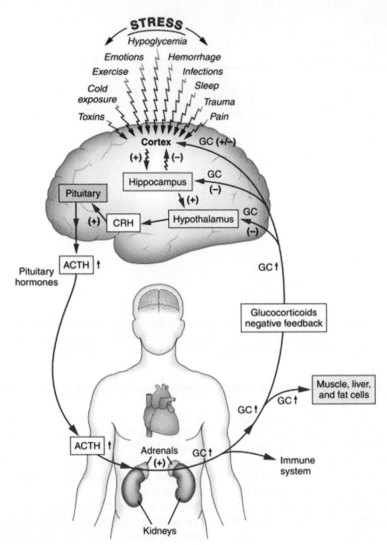

Fig. 4. Normal hypothalamic-pituitary-adrenal axis involved in glucocorticoid production. (*From* Norman AW, Henry HL. Adrenal corticoids. [Chapter 10]. In: Hormones. 3rd edition. Academic Press; 2015. p. 230; with permission.)

upper limit of normal. In nonclassic CAH, the baseline 17-OHP level may be normal to mildly elevated.[1]

The recommended diagnostic procedure for all forms of CAH is the 60-minute ACTH (cosyntropin) stimulation test. The test is performed in early morning (8 AM), when cortisol secretion is at its normal diurnal peak. A complete adrenocortical profile (including aldosterone and renin levels) is obtained before and then 60 minutes after administration of a 0.25-mg intravenous or intramuscular bolus of ACTH. The 17-OHP level is markedly elevated following ACTH administration in the classic and non-classic forms of 21-hydroxylase deficiency.[1,6]

Treatment

Treatment for CAH involves replacement of the deficient hormones. Glucocorticoid therapy replaces deficient cortisol to prevent adrenal crisis, which helps normalize the excessive, adrenal androgen production.[1] Hydrocortisone is the preferred corticosteroid in children with all forms of CAH because its short half-life minimizes potential side effects of longer-acting glucocorticoids.[6] The 2010 Endocrine Society guidelines recommend that all patients with classic CAH receive fludrocortisone (Florinef) and sodium chloride supplementation during the newborn period and early infancy.[6]

Recombinant human growth hormone can either be used alone or in combination with a gonadotropin-releasing hormone analogue to improve final adult height in patients with CAH.[1] Management of ambiguous genitalia is handled with genital surgery.[6]

ADRENAL INSUFFICIENCY
Background

Adrenal insufficiency results from failure of the adrenal cortex to produce sufficient steroid hormones. Primary adrenal insufficiency (Addison disease) is caused by diseases that affect the adrenal cortex and is uncommon, with an incidence of 4 to 6 in 1 million per year. Primary adrenal insufficiency is characterized by low cortisol, low aldosterone, and high CRH and ACTH levels.[1] Secondary adrenal insufficiency is more common and is characterized by low cortisol and low CRH and ACTH levels.[1] This article mostly discusses primary adrenal insufficiency.

Causes of primary adrenal insufficiency are classified into infectious, autoimmune, and genetic disorders. The most frequent cause of primary adrenal insufficiency worldwide is tuberculosis. In developed countries, 80% to 90% of patients with primary adrenal insufficiency have an autoimmune cause where the 21-hydroxylase enzyme is most frequently targeted by autoantibodies. For a full list of causes of primary and secondary adrenal insufficiency see **Box 1**.[1,7]

Clinical Features

Onset of fulminant disease is often gradual in primary adrenal insufficiency and approximately 50% of patients have symptoms greater than 1 year before diagnosis. Symptoms include weakness, fatigue, nausea, vomiting, anorexia, diarrhea, abdominal pain, weight loss, salt craving, and orthostasis. Hyperpigmentation of skin, mucosa, hair, and nails only occurs in primary adrenal insufficiency as a result of elevated ACTH and melanocyte-stimulating hormone levels, which stimulate melanocortin-1 receptors on cutaneous melanocytes.[1] Other signs of adrenal insufficiency include shock; hypotension; weight loss; and electrolyte abnormalities, such as hyponatremia, hyperkalemia, metabolic acidosis, and hypoglycemia (**Fig. 5**).[7]

Diagnosis

Synthetic ACTH testing, also known as cosyntropin (Cortrosyn) stimulation, has become the gold standard screening test for diagnosis of primary adrenal insufficiency.[7] The test is quick, not affected by diet or medication, simple to interpret, and can be applied to people of all ages.[1] In adults and children greater than or equal to 2 years old, synthetic ACTH 250 µg is administered intravenously at any time of day and blood samples measuring cortisol levels are drawn at 0, 30, and 60 minutes. Cortisol values less than 18 µg/dL either at 30 or 60 minutes indicate adrenal insufficiency.[7] Baseline measurement of plasma ACTH, aldosterone, and plasma renin activity (PRA) at time 0 (before the administration of cosyntropin) is advised. In

Box 1
Causes of primary and secondary adrenal insufficiency

Causes of Primary Adrenal Insufficiency

Autoimmune
  Autoimmune Addison disease
  Autoimmune polyendocrinopathy syndrome type I
  Autoimmune polyendocrinopathy syndrome type II
  X-linked polyendocrinopathy

Infectious
  Tuberculosis
  Fungal: histoplasmosis, blastomycosis, coccidioidomycosis, cryptococcosis
  AIDS with opportunistic infections, such as cytomegalovirus, mycobacterium, fungi, Kaposi
  sarcoma

Adrenal infiltration
  Metastasis from breast, lung, stomach, and colon cancer
  Lymphomas
  Amyloidosis
  Sarcoidosis
  Hemochromatosis

Bilateral adrenalectomy

Bilateral adrenal hemorrhage or infarction

Medications
  Etomidate, mitotane, ketoconazole

Genetic disorders
  Congenital adrenal hyperplasia
  Congenital lipoid adrenal hyperplasia
  Adrenoleukodystrophy and adrenomyeloneuropathy, also known as Brown Schilder disease
  Familial glucocorticoid deficiency type 1, type 2, or type 3
  Triple A syndrome (Allgrove syndrome)
  Congenital adrenal hypoplasia

Causes of Secondary Adrenal Insufficiency

Hypothalamic-pituitary-adrenal suppression
  Exogenous glucocorticoid administration
    Oral, topical, or inhaled steroids

Tumors/destruction of hypothalamus or pituitary
  Pituitary tumors
  Metastatic tumors
  Amyloidosis
  Sarcoidosis
  Craniopharyngiomas
  Rathke pouch cysts
  Head trauma

Infections affecting the hypothalamus or pituitary
  Tuberculosis
  Actinomyosis
  Nocardiosis

Vascular accidents
  Sheehan syndrome

Isolated deficiency of ACTH

Autoimmune
  Autoimmune lymphocytic hypophysitis

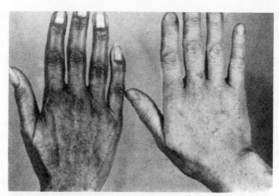

Fig. 5. Hyperpigmentation associated with primary adrenal insufficiency. The hand on the left is from a patient with Addison disease. The hand on the right is from a healthy individual. (*From* Norman AW, Henry HL. Adrenal corticoids. [Chapter 10]. In: Hormones. 3rd edition. Academic Press; 2015. p. 236)

patients with cortisol deficiency, a plasma ACTH greater than two-fold the upper limit of the reference range is consistent with primary adrenal insufficiency.[7]

Antibodies against 21-hydroxylase are tested if autoimmune adrenal insufficiency is suspected. In patients with suspected adrenal hemorrhage, infection, infiltration, or neoplastic disease, abdominal computed tomography (CT) should be performed.[1]

Treatment

Treatment of adrenal insufficiency consists of replacing the missing steroid hormones: cortisol and aldosterone in primary adrenal insufficiency and cortisol alone in secondary adrenal insufficiency. Either hydrocortisone, 15 to 25 mg/day, or cortisone acetate, 20 to 35 mg/day, in two or three divided doses is recommended for cortisol replacement. Monitoring of glucocorticoid replacement should be through clinical assessment of blood pressure, energy, body weight, and signs of glucocorticoid excess.[7] All patients with aldosterone deficiency should receive fludrocortisone (Florinef), which is normally given as a single daily dose of 50 to 200 μg/day along with unrestricted salt intake. Response to mineralocorticoid replacement with fludrocortisone is primarily through clinical assessment of blood pressure, edema, salt craving, and electrolyte measurements.[1,7]

Approximately 90% of DHEA and DHEA-S originates from the adrenal gland and in women with adrenal insufficiency, the reduction in DHEA and DHEA-S production results in androgen deficiency. Recent Endocrine Society practice guidelines from 2016 recommend a 6-month trial of DHEA replacement in women with primary adrenal insufficiency and reduced libido, depressive symptoms, and low energy despite optimized glucocorticoid and mineralocorticoid replacement.[7]

During minor stresses, such as febrile illness, minor surgical procedures, such as dental work, and minor trauma, such as lacerations and contusion, the steroid dose should be doubled. Adults with suspected adrenal crisis should be given an immediate parenteral injection of 100 mg hydrocortisone (50 mg/m² for children) followed by fluid resuscitation and 200 mg of hydrocortisone/24 hours (50–100 mg/m² for children).[7]

Patients with adrenal insufficiency should understand how to manage their condition, including glucocorticoid adjustments during stress and adrenal crisis. It is also recommended that patients always carry a medical alert card, necklace, or bracelet denoting their diagnosis, medications, and emergency plan. A hydrocortisone emergency injection kit consisting of a vial of 100 mg hydrocortisone, a syringe, and needle should also be prescribed for urgent administration during adrenal crisis, especially in the presence of vomiting and/or diarrhea. This is particularly useful if patients travel to places where there is less familiarity with their diagnosis or if the patient will be in a remote area (ie, camping or hiking).[7]

ADRENAL CAUSES OF HYPERCORTISOLISM
Background

Chronic glucocorticoid excess can result from many causes and is termed Cushing syndrome, irrespective of the cause. The most common cause of glucocorticoid excess is from medically prescribed, exogenous corticosteroids.[8] Endogenous hypercortisolism is much less common with an incidence of 2 to 10 patients per million per year.[1,8] Excessive cortisol production can result from either inappropriate secretion of ACTH by pituitary or ectopic sources or from adrenal cortisol overproduction, independent of ACTH levels.[9] Approximately 80% of cases of endogenous hypercortisolism result from an ACTH-secreting pituitary adenoma.[8,9] Although uncommon, this article focuses mainly on ACTH-independent adrenal causes of Cushing syndrome as summarized in **Box 2**.[1,8]

Adrenal lesions responsible for Cushing syndrome typically arise from the zona fasciculata within the adrenal cortex. Benign adenomas are the most common cause of adrenal Cushing in adult patients (50%–80%), followed by adrenal cortex carcinoma (20%), then followed by adrenal hyperplasia (10%–15%).[1,8] In children, adrenal cortex carcinoma accounts for a larger share of Cushing cases, with the remainder caused by either adenomas or genetic conditions, such as primary pigmented nodular adrenal dysplasia or McCune-Albright syndrome.[1] Patients with persistent hypercortisolism have a 3.8-fold to five-fold increased risk of mortality compared with the general population.[10]

Clinical Features

Clinical features of hypercortisolism vary according to the extent and duration of hypercortisolism and include obesity, hypertension, proximal muscle wasting, a rounded erythematous face, acne, hirsutism, supraclavicular fat pads, dorsocervical fat accumulation ("buffalo hump"), purple striae, easy bruising, skin thinning, reduced bone density, pathologic fractures, menstrual irregularities, reduced libido or impotence, fatigue, insomnia, psychiatric alterations ranging from irritability to mania, increased white blood cell count, a slightly elevated red blood cell count, increased low-density lipoprotein and triglycerides, cardiovascular disease, and impaired glucose tolerance.[8,10] Children may present with stunted height velocity and increased weight gain.[9] Electrolyte imbalances, such as hypokalemia, are more common in severe hypercortisolism.[1] Adrenal cortex carcinoma may present with mass-related signs, symptoms of metastatic disease, or nonspecific features of malignancy, such as weight loss, fever, and anorexia.[1] In subclinical Cushing syndrome there may

---

Box 2
ACTH-independent adrenal causes of Cushing syndrome

Tumors arising from the zona fasciculata of the adrenal cortex, either benign or carcinoma

ACTH-independent adrenal hyperplasia, either macronodular or micronodular

Primary pigmented nodular adrenal dysplasia, either sporadic or familial as part of the Carney complex

McCune-Albright syndrome

be no clinically apparent signs or symptoms of hypercortisolism in the setting of autonomous cortisol secretion, such as in an incidentally found adrenal mass on imaging performed for unrelated disease (**Fig. 6**).[11]

Diagnosis

Diagnosis of Cushing syndrome is made by careful testing of urine, saliva, and/or blood cortisol levels taking into account individual patient comorbidities, medication use, and lifestyle characteristics that can affect interpretation of test results. Distinguishing Cushing syndrome from a pseudo-Cushing state is difficult because psychiatric conditions, obesity, alcoholism, and diabetes result in overactivation of the hypothalamic-pituitary-adrenal axis without true Cushing syndrome.[8] Work-up for Cushing syndrome typically yields inconsistent results and no laboratory test or imaging study is 100% diagnostic.

After excluding exogenous steroid use as a cause of hypercortisolism, the Endocrine Society guidelines recommend one of the following initial tests for Cushing syndrome: at least two separate measurements of 24-hour urine free cortisol or late night

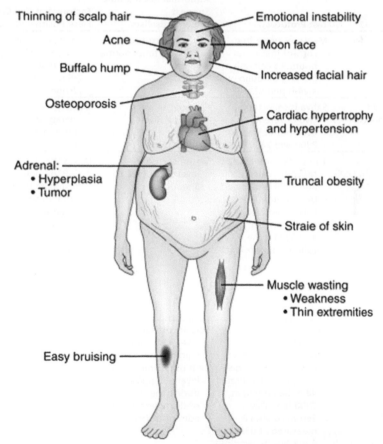

Fig. 6. Clinical manifestations of Cushing syndrome in a female. (*From* Norman AW, Henry HL. Adrenal corticoids. [Chapter 10]. In: Hormones. 3rd edition. Academic Press; 2015. p. 234; with permission.)

salivary cortisol, 1 mg overnight dexamethasone suppression test, or longer low-dose dexamethasone suppression test.[9,10] These tests evaluate for loss of the normal circadian rhythm of cortisol secretion and are summarized in **Table 1**.[8–10]

If results of initial cortisol testing suggest hypercortisolism, then the next step is to determine whether ACTH-dependent or ACTH-independent disease is present by measuring plasma ACTH levels. In adrenal Cushing the plasma ACTH is typically suppressed (<10 pg/mL), whereas the ACTH level is normal or increased in ACTH-dependent forms of Cushing.[8]

If ACTH-dependent Cushing syndrome is suspected, then a pituitary MRI with gadolinium should be performed. Bilateral inferior petrosal sinus sampling is considered the gold standard for establishing the origin of ACTH secretion and is recommended in patients with ACTH-dependent Cushing whose clinical, biochemical, or radiologic findings are discordant or in patients with a negative pituitary MRI who have

Table 1
Initial tests used to diagnose Cushing syndrome

Test Name	Test Protocol	Abnormal Results that Suggest Hypercortisolism	Factors that Can Cause False-Positive Results
24-h urine free cortisol	Measures urine free cortisol that is not bound to cortisol-binding globulin over a 24-h period.	Urine free cortisol levels >4 times normal range	Obesity, depression, anxiety, diabetes, high fluid intake ≥5 L/d, and alcoholism.
Late night salivary cortisol	Saliva is collected on two different evenings between 2300 and 2400 h.	Elevated salivary cortisol levels between 2300 and 2400 h.	Obesity, depression, anxiety, diabetes, shift work, licorice, chewing tobacco.
1-mg overnight DST	1-mg dexamethasone is taken between 2300 and 2400 h followed by measurement of cortisol and ACTH levels between 0800 and 0900 h the following morning.	Serum cortisol level >1.8 µg/dL to 5 µg/dL.	Drugs that induce CYP3A4 hepatic dexamethasone metabolism (alcohol, barbiturates, phenytoin, carbamazepine, rifampicin), impaired dexamethasone absorption, liver or renal failure, estrogen treatment, and pseudo-Cushing.
48 h, 2 mg low-dose DST	In adults and children >40 kg, dexamethasone is given in 0.5-mg doses every 6 h for a total of 48 h, beginning at 0900 h on Day 1. Serum cortisol is measured at 0900 h, 6 h after the last dose of dexamethasone.	Serum cortisol level >1.8 µg/dL to 5 µg/dL. 24-h urine free cortisol level >10 µg/24 h during the second day of dexamethasone administration.	Same factors as for the 1-mg overnight DST

DST, dexamethasone suppression test.

biochemical evidence of hypercortisolism.[8] A ratio of central to peripheral ACTH greater than two in the basal state or greater than three after CRH stimulation is consistent with pituitary Cushing disease.[8] If bilateral inferior petrosal sinus sampling does not show a central gradient, then CT and/or MRI scans of the neck/chest, abdomen, and pelvis should be performed to evaluate for an ectopic source of ACTH secretion.[8]

If ACTH-independent Cushing syndrome is suspected, then adrenal CT or MRI should be performed to identify the type of adrenal lesion. Abnormal results from adrenal imaging must be interpreted with caution because of the high prevalence of adrenal incidentaloma in the general population (up to 5%), making it difficult to distinguish between abnormal imaging findings caused by a nonfunctioning incidentaloma versus a pathologic adrenal lesion.[8]

Treatment

High morbidity and mortality occurs in Cushing syndrome mainly because of cardiovascular disease and comorbidities, such as hypertension, diabetes, dyslipidemia, infections, osteoporosis, and a hypercoagulable state. Management of cardiovascular risk factors and comorbid conditions is crucial.[12]

Endocrine Society guidelines from 2015 recommend surgical resection of the primary lesions causing Cushing syndrome as a first-line treatment strategy whenever possible.[12] Transsphenoidal selective adenomectomy is the optimal treatment of pituitary Cushing disease.[12] Surgical removal of an adrenal adenoma occurs by either partial or total unilateral adrenalectomy and usually results in remission of hypercortisolism. Adrenal insufficiency may occur after removal of hyperfunctioning adrenal tissue requiring steroid replacement that may be gradually tapered over time depending on recovery of the hypothalamic-pituitary-adrenal axis. Surveillance is necessary after surgical removal of both pituitary and adrenal adenomas because Cushing syndrome may recur.[1,12]

Drugs to control hypercortisolism may be used either in preparation for surgery, if surgery is unsuccessful, or in patients who are not surgical candidates and are classified into four groups: (1) adrenolytic, (2) adrenostatic, (3) glucocorticoid receptor antagonist, and (4) somatostatin analogues (**Box 3**).[1,12]

PRIMARY ALDOSTERONISM (CONN SYNDROME)
Background

Aldosterone is the most important mineralocorticoid hormone and is synthesized in the zona glomerulosa. Aldosterone causes sodium reabsorption by the renal cortical collecting duct in exchange for potassium and hydrogen ion excretion into urine, leading to increased extracellular fluid volume and suppressed renin secretion.[1]

Primary aldosteronism involves inappropriately increased aldosterone secretion that is autonomous and independent of the renin-angiotensin system and is nonsuppressible by sodium loading.[13] Secondary aldosteronism refers to disorders in which aldosterone excess results from overactivation of the renin-angiotensin system.[1] This article focuses on primary hyperaldosteronism (**Box 4**).

Clinical Features

Inappropriate production of aldosterone can lead to cardiovascular disease, suppressed plasma renin, hypertension, sodium retention, and hypokalemia. All patients with hypertension and hypokalemia (spontaneous or diuretic-induced) should be screened for aldosteronism in addition to patients with early onset cerebrovascular

---

Box 3
Drugs used to control hypercortisolism

Adrenolytic drugs: destroys adrenocortical cells and reduces steroid synthesis; mostly used in adrenocortical cancer.
  Mitotane: starting dose 0.5 to 2 g/day and the dose is increased by 1 g every 4 weeks up to a maximal daily dose of 4 to 12 g.

Adrenostatic drugs: interferes with steroidogenesis without damaging adrenal cells; can be used in all forms of Cushing syndrome.
  Ketoconazole: starting dose 200 mg/day and progressively increased to 600 to 800 mg/day according to adrenal secretory parameters.
  Metyrapone: doses range from 500 mg/day to 6 g/day, divided in 3 to 4 doses.
  Etomidate: given intravenously 1.2 to 2.5 mg/h; only indicated to reduce hypercortisolism in severely ill patients who are not responsive or nothing-by-mouth.
  Trilostane

Glucocorticoid receptor antagonist: reduces symptoms of hypercortisolism by competitively binding glucocorticoid and progesterone receptors, blocking peripheral effects of excess steroids.
  Mifepristone (RU-486): doses range from 300 to 1200 mg/day.

Somatostatin analogues: binds to somatostatin receptors and blocks release of ACTH.
  Pasireotide: starting dose is 0.6 mg subcutaneously twice daily and may be increased to 0.9 mg twice daily.

Data from Jameson JL, De Groot LJ, Kretser DM. Endocrinology: adult & pediatric, vol. II. 7th edition. Philadelphia: Elsevier; 2016. p. 1785–930; and Nieman LK, Biller BM, Findling JW, et al. Treatment of Cushing's syndrome: an Endocrine Society Clinical Practice Guideline. J Clin Endocrinol Metab 2015;100(8):2807–31.

---

accident before age 40, a family history of early stroke in a first-degree relative, adrenal incidentalomas and hypertension, and difficult to control blood pressure despite use of three antihypertensive agents from different drug classes.[13]

Diagnosis

The diagnosis of primary aldosteronism should be distinguished from administration of exogenous mineralocorticoids (ie, fludrocortisone), licorice ingestion, or secretion of excess mineralocorticoids other than aldosterone (ie, deoxycorticosterone associated with 17a-hydroxylase deficiency).[1]

To screen for primary aldosteronism, a morning blood sample is collected for PRA and plasma aldosterone concentration (PAC). The test may be performed while the patient is taking antihypertensive medications except for spironolactone, eplerenone, and amiloride. If the PAC/PRA ratio is greater than or equal to 30 (with PAC expressed as ng/dL and PRA as ng/mL/h) then further investigation for primary aldosteronism should occur.[1]

A variety of factors can affect PAC/PRA ratio results. False-positive results can occur in renal impairment, use of β-blockers, nonsteroidal anti-inflammatory drug use, and advanced age by causing renin suppression. False-negative results can occur with hypokalemia, sodium restriction (which increases renin production), use of diuretics, angiotensin-converting enzyme inhibitors, angiotensin receptor blockers, aldosterone blockers, and dihydropyridine calcium channel blockers.[1]

A positive PAC/PRA ratio screening test should prompt further investigation with one of four aldosterone suppression tests (**Table 2**) to confirm the diagnosis before subtype classification. Three of the tests are salt-loading tests: in normal subjects volume expansion with saline suppresses plasma aldosterone, whereas volume

> **Box 4**
> **Forms of primary aldosteronism (listed in order of prevalence)**
>
> Bilateral idiopathic adrenal hyperplasia
>
> Aldosterone-producing adenoma
>
> Primary (unilateral) adrenal hyperplasia
>
> Aldosterone-producing adrenocortical carcinoma
>
> Ectopic (nonadrenal) aldosterone-producing adenoma
>
> Familial hyperaldosteronism
>   Type I: glucocorticoid-remediable hyperaldosteronism
>   Type II: can present with either aldosterone-producing adenoma or bilateral idiopathic
>   adrenal hyperplasia
>   Type III: involves massive adrenal hyperplasia in childhood
>
> *Data from* Jameson JL, De Groot LJ, Kretser DM. Endocrinology: adult & pediatric, vol. II. 7th
> edition. Philadelphia: Elsevier; 2016. p. 1785–930.

expansion in primary aldosteronism does not exert the same suppressive action on aldosterone secretion. The fourth test depends on inhibition of aldosterone secretion by an angiotensin-converting enzyme inhibitor.[13]

After the diagnosis of primary aldosteronism has been confirmed using one of the previously mentioned tests, unilateral disease (usually resulting from an aldosterone producing adenoma) needs to be differentiated from bilateral disease (usually resulting from adrenal hyperplasia), aldosterone-producing carcinoma, and extremely rare tumors causing ectopic aldosterone production.[1]

An adrenal CT scan is recommended to evaluate the appearance of the adrenal glands and to exclude large masses that may represent adrenocortical carcinoma. Adrenal vein sampling is used to differentiate unilateral from bilateral disease.[13]

Treatment

Patients with unilateral disease (aldosterone-producing adenoma and unilateral adrenal hyperplasia) should receive unilateral adrenalectomy, whereas medical treatments with aldosterone antagonists (ie, spironolactone or eplerenone) and/or other drugs (ie, amiloride) are used in bilateral disease.[13]

PHEOCHROMOCYTOMA
Background

A pheochromocytoma is a tumor arising from adrenal medullary chromaffin tissue that produces one or more catecholamines: epinephrine, norepinephrine, and dopamine. A paraganglioma is a tumor arising from extra-adrenal sympathetic or parasympathetic ganglia.[14] Incidence is 3 to 8 cases per 1 million per year in the general population, most commonly occurring during the fourth and fifth decades and occurring equally in men and women. Most pheochromocytomas arise sporadically but up to 35% are inherited associated with multiple endocrine neoplasia type 2, von Hippel-Lindau disease, neurofibromatosis type 1, and familial paraganglioma.[1]

Clinical Features

Signs and symptoms of pheochromocytoma result from hemodynamic and metabolic consequences of excess circulating catecholamines and metanephrines, leading to high morbidity and mortality.[14]

Table 2
Summary of confirmation tests for diagnosis of primary aldosteronism

Test Name	Test Protocol	Normal Results	Abnormal Results that Suggest Primary Aldosteronism
Oral sodium loading test	Increase dietary sodium intake to 300 mmol/d × 3 d and verify by 24-h urine sodium excretion. Give slow-release KCl to maintain normokalemia.	Urine aldosterone secretion ≤12 mg/24 h	Urine aldosterone secretion >12 mg/24 h
Intravenous saline suppression test	2 L normal saline intravenously over 4 h. Measure PAC at baseline and at 4 h.	PAC <5 ng/dL at 4 h Intermediate result is PAC 5–10 ng/dL at 4 h	PAC ≥15 ng/dL at baseline and ≥10 ng/dL at 4 h
Fludrocortisone suppression test	4 d of a high sodium diet + slow release NaCl 30 mEq TID + fludrocortisone 100 μg q 6 h	PAC ≤6 ng/dL on Day 4 (upright, 10 AM)	PAC >6 ng/dL on Day 4 (upright, 10 AM)
Captopril challenge test	Administer captopril 25–50 mg orally in a seated patient and measure plasma aldosterone levels 2 h later	Suppression of PAC by 30% from baseline	Absence of suppression of PAC by 30% from baseline

Data from Jameson JL, De Groot LJ, Kretser DM. Endocrinology: adult & pediatric, vol. II. 7th edition. Philadelphia: Elsevier; 2016. p. 1785–930; and Funder JW, Carey RM, Fardella C, et al. Case detection, diagnosis, and treatment of patients with primary aldosteronism: an Endocrine Society Clinical Practice Guideline. J Clin Endocrinol Metab 2008;93(9):3266–81.

Clinical findings include hypertension, headache, unusual sweating, arrhythmias/palpitations, pallor during hypertensive episodes, abdominal pain, anxiety, weight loss (caused by catecholamine-induced glycogenolysis and lipolysis), and generalized weakness. The triad of headache, diaphoresis, and tachycardia, especially in the setting of either sustained or paroxysmal hypertension should raise suspicion for a pheochromocytoma.[15]

The clinical presentation of pheochromocytoma can be variable, with similar signs and symptoms produced by multiple other conditions including thyrotoxicosis; cardiovascular disease; migraine or cluster headaches; anxiety attacks; medullary thyroid carcinoma; carcinoid syndrome; hypoglycemia; menopause; porphyria; illicit drugs, such as amphetamines and cocaine; and ingestion of tyramine-containing foods or over-the-counter sympathomimetics (ie, Sudafed) especially in combination with taking monoamine oxidase inhibitors (**Fig. 7**).[1]

Diagnosis

Measurements of urinary or plasma catecholamines can be unreliable for detecting a pheochromocytoma, because catecholamine secretion can be episodic. Normetanephrine and metanephrine (collectively referred to as metanephrines) are metabolites of the catecholamines (norepinephrine and epinephrine), respectively, and are more consistently elevated in the setting of pheochromocytoma than their parent

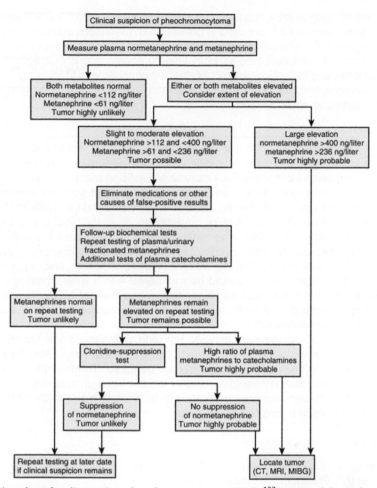

Fig. 7. Flowchart for diagnosing pheochromocytoma. MIBG, ^{123}I-metaiodobenzylguanidine.

catecholamines. As a result, initial biochemical testing for pheochromocytoma and paraganglioma should include measurements of plasma free metanephrines (with patients in the supine position for 30 minutes before the laboratory draw) and/or urinary fractionated metanephrines over a 24-hour period.[14]

Medications that can cause false-positive elevations of plasma and urinary metanephrine and catecholamine levels include acetaminophen, selective serotonin reuptake inhibitors, tricyclic antidepressants, α- and β-adrenergic blockers, calcium channel blockers, monoamine oxidase inhibitors, ephedrine, pseudoephedrine, albuterol, caffeine, levodopa, carbidopa, hydralazine, and minoxidil.[1,14,15] These medications should be discontinued for 10 to 14 days before testing if possible.[15]

Localization of pheochromocytoma with CT, MRI, and/or functional imaging studies should be performed only if clinical and biochemical findings are reasonably compelling. Approximately 80% of tumors are located in the adrenal glands.[1] Because extra-adrenal pheochromocytomas are most commonly located in the abdomen, CT of the abdomen/pelvis should be performed first followed by chest and neck imaging if abdominal CT is negative.[14] MRI is indicated in patients with metastatic disease.[14]

Functional imaging studies, including ^{123}I-metaiodobenzylguanidine scintigraphy and ^{18}F-fluorodeoxyglucose PET, are used in patients with metastatic pheochromocytoma or paraganglioma.[14] It should be noted that metastatic pheochromocytoma may undergo tumor dedifferentiation leading to inability to accumulate pheochromocytoma-specific isotopes and lack of localization. Metastatic pheochromocytomas may express somatostatin receptors, thus enabling somatostatin receptor scintigraphy with the somatostatin analogue octreotide (Octreoscan).

Treatment

Treatment of pheochromocytoma involves prompt surgical removal of the tumor, because catecholamine excess is associated with significant mortality rates of 45%.[14,15] Preoperative considerations include normalizing blood pressure and heart rate, correcting volume depletion, and preventing a patient from surgery-induced catecholamine storm. α-Adrenergic blockers, dihydropyridine calcium channel blockers, metyrosine (Desmer), and/or angiotensin receptor blockers are recommended preoperatively to avoid hypertensive crisis.[14,15] β-Blockers should not be used to control tachycardia until a patient is fully α-blocked to prevent unopposed α-adrenergic stimulation leading to severe vasoconstriction and hypertensive crisis.[15] Plasma metanephrines should be monitored 4 to 8 weeks postoperatively to ensure successful removal of all tumor tissue and then at least once annually for life given the potential for multiple primary tumors, recurrence, and the long latency for metastatic disease.[15]

Approximately 25% of pheochromocytomas and paragangliomas are malignant with either local invasion into adjacent tissue or distant metastases. Unless full surgical resection is possible, metastatic disease cannot be cured. Treatments with chemotherapy, ^{123}I-metaiodobenzylguanidine, and/or radiation can provide disease control. α-Blockade is necessary during any treatment to prevent hypertensive crisis from catecholamine release during tumor cell lysis.[15]

REFERENCES

1. Jameson JL, De Groot LJ, Kretser DM. 7th edition. Endocrinology: adult & pediatric, vol. II. Philadelphia: Elsevier; 2016. p. 1785–930.
2. Vrezas I, Willenberg HS, Bornstein SR. Adrenal cortex, anatomy. In: Martini L, editor. Encyclopedia of endocrine diseases, vol. I, 1st edition. Amsterdam: Academic Press; 2004. p. 50–2.
3. Norman AW, Henry HL. Adrenal corticoids [Chapter 10]. In: Hormones. 3rd edition. London, UK: Academic Press; 2015. p. 223–38.
4. Nicolaides NC, Charmandari E, Chrousos GP. Adrenal steroid hormone secretion: physiologic and endocrine aspects. In: Caplan MJ, editor. Reference module in biomedical sciences. 3rd edition. 2014. p. 1–7.
5. Turcu AF, Auchus RJ. Adrenal steroidogenesis and congenital adrenal hyperplasia. Endocrinol Metab Clin N Am 2015;44(2):275–96.
6. Speiser PW, Azziz R, Baskin LS, et al. Congenital adrenal hyperplasia due to steroid 21-hydroxylase deficiency: an endocrine society clinical practice guideline. J Clin Endocrinol Metab 2010;95(9):4133–60.
7. Bornstein SR, Allolio B, Arlt B, et al. Diagnosis and treatment of primary adrenal insufficiency: an endocrine society clinical practice guideline. J Clin Endocrinol Metab 2016;101(2):364–89.
8. Boscaro M, Arnaldi G. Approach to the patient with possible Cushing's syndrome. J Clin Endocrinol Metab 2009;94(9):3121–31.

9. Nieman LK, Biller BM, Findling JW, et al. The diagnosis of Cushing's syndrome: an endocrine society clinical practice guideline. J Clin Endocrinol Metab 2008; 93(5):1526–40.
10. Carroll TB, Findling JW. The diagnosis of Cushing's syndrome. Rev Endocr Metab Disord 2010;11:147–53.
11. De Leo M, Cozzolino A, Colao A, et al. Subclinical Cushing's syndrome. Best Pract Res Clin Endocrinol Metab 2012;26(4):497–505.
12. Nieman LK, Biller BM, Findling JW, et al. Treatment of Cushing's syndrome: an endocrine society clinical practice guideline. J Clin Endocrinol Metab 2015; 100(8):2807–31.
13. Funder JW, Carey RM, Fardella C, et al. Case detection, diagnosis, and treatment of patients with primary aldosteronism: an endocrine society clinical practice guideline. J Clin Endocrinol Metab 2008;93(9):3266–81.
14. Lenders JW, Duh QY, Eisenhofer G. Pheochromocytoma and paraganglioma: an endocrine society clinical practice guideline. J Clin Endocrinol Metab 2014;99(6): 1915–42.
15. Fishbein L. Pheochromocytoma and paraganglioma: genetics, diagnosis, and treatment. Hematol Oncol Clin N Am 2016;30(1):135–50.

Misconceptions in Evaluation and Treatment of Calcium Abnormalities and Parathyroid Disorders

Ashlyn Smith, MMS, PA-C

KEYWORDS

- Calcium • Hypercalcemia • Hypocalcemia • Parathyroid • Hyperparathyroidism
- Hypoparathyroidism • Adenoma

KEY POINTS

- The treatment goal for hypocalcemia secondary to hypoparathyroidism is low-normal to marginally low serum calcium with normal 24-hour urine calcium.
- Normal intact parathyroid hormone in the presence of hypercalcemia is not physiologic and does not rule out primary hyperparathyroidism (PHPT).
- Localization (imaging) studies are used to aid preoperative mapping for parathyroidectomy rather than required to make the diagnosis of PHTP.
- Parathyroidectomy is the recommended intervention for PHPT in patients who meet surgical criteria.

EPIDEMIOLOGY

Eucalcemia is essential for multiple physiologic processes, including nerve conduction, muscle contraction, and bone strength. Even mild abnormalities in serum calcium levels may be pathologic and should be investigated. Primary hyperparathyroidism (PHPT) is most often the cause of outpatient hypercalcemia and is present in about 1% of the adult population.[1] PHPT is 2 to 3 times more common in women and is most often caused by a single parathyroid adenoma.[1] Conversely, hypocalcemia secondary to hypoparathyroidism is the most common complication after thyroidectomy after inadvertent removal or damage to one or more of the parathyroid glands.[2,3] However, the actual incidence of postoperative hypoparathyroidism is not well determined due to a discordance of criteria to define these cases.[2] This review explores the manifestation, pathophysiology, causes, evaluation, and treatment of calcium disorders.

Disclosure: The author has nothing to disclose.
Endocrinology Associates, Scottsdale, Arizona, USA
E-mail address: ashlyns9@endoassocaz.net

Physician Assist Clin 2 (2017) 141–153
http://dx.doi.org/10.1016/j.cpha.2016.08.011
2405-7991/17/© 2016 Elsevier Inc. All rights reserved.

In particular, this review delineates common misconceptions in the evaluation and treatment of calcium disorders and describes the appropriate alternatives.

CALCIUM METABOLISM

Calcium balance is maintained by a harmony between gut absorption, renal reabsorption, and bone matrix turnover.[4] In response to decreased serum calcium, parathyroid hormone (PTH) is released, which stimulates both renal tubular reabsorption and bone calcium resorption.[4] In addition, PTH promotes hydroxylation of 25-hydroxyvitamin D to 1,25-dihydroxyvitamin D (the most active form of vitamin D) from the kidney, which allows for increased intestinal calcium absorption and bone resorption.[4] Finally, 1,25-dihydroxyvitamin D provides negative feedback to the parathyroid glands to decrease PTH secretion.[4]

Conversely, elevated serum calcium levels suppress PTH release; this limits renal tubular reabsorption, bone calcium resorption, and 1,25-dihydroxyvitamin D production. Lower 1,25-dihydroxyvitamin D further decreases bone resorption as well as intestinal calcium absorption. This confluence of events results in a net decrease in serum calcium in an effort to reinstate normocalcemia.

HYPOCALCEMIA

Whether hypocalcemia is found incidentally on comprehensive or basic metabolic panel or during a diagnostic evaluation, an investigation for clinical manifestations is prudent. Patients may be asymptomatic or may report muscle cramping or tingling to the perioral region, hands, or feet.[2] On examination, there may be no clinical manifestations. However, in severe hypocalcemia, positive Chvostek and Trousseau signs may be present[2]: positive Chvostek sign is a provoked twitching or spasm in the ipsilateral facial muscle by stimulating the facial nerve (tapping the masseter muscle anterior to the jaw angle); positive Trousseau sign is observing carpopedal spasm on inflation of sphygmomanometer on the ipsilateral arm for 3 minutes (**Figs. 1** and **2**).

Although Chvostek and Trousseau signs are pathognomonic for hypocalcemia, hyperesthesias may be attributed to other conditions, including but not limited to, neuropathy, multiple sclerosis, and anxiety. Clinical judgment should be used when interpreting the relevancy of the symptoms. If the symptoms seem out of proportion to the level of hypocalcemia or persist after correction, other causes should be investigated.

Diagnostic Approach

Once hypocalcemia is detected, the first step is to confirm the abnormal finding and is done by assessing serum calcium levels in the context of albumin[3] using the equation corrected calcium = serum calcium + 0.8 × (4 − serum albumin). Ionized calcium, or the measurement of biochemically active calcium, is useful if hypocalcemia is suspected based on history and symptoms, but total serum calcium is within normal limits (and vice versa). After confirming hypocalcemia, the next studies should be targeted at assessing for the most common cause: parathyroid disease. This assessment is done using measures of intact PTH (iPTH) as well as assessing levels that can affect the interpretation of iPTH with 25-hydroxyvitamin D level, renal functions, phosphorus, and magnesium.[3] Assessment for underlying hypomagnesemia should be considered and corrected because low magnesium levels will limit calcium absorption because of PTH resistance.[2]

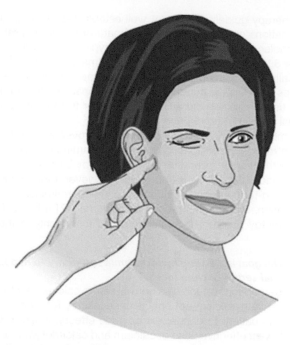

Fig. 1. Chvostek sign. *From* Carlson K. AACN Advanced Critical Care Nursing. Philadelphia, PA: Elsevier;2009. p. 841–64;with permission.

Therapeutic Goals

Treatment of hypocalcemia secondary to hypoparathyroidism is with over-the-counter calcium and prescription calcitriol.[2] Calcitriol is preferred over cholecalciferol due to the shorter half-life, which allows for quicker reversal of damaging vitamin D toxicity. Initial starting treatment doses are elemental calcium 1000 mg 3 times daily and calcitriol 0.5 mg twice daily.[2] In the presence of hypomagnesemia and normal renal function, replacement with magnesium oxide 400 mg twice daily is recommended.[2] Life-threatening hypocalcemia requires emergency replacement, which is not covered in this review.

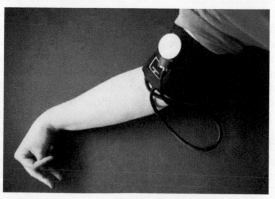

Fig. 2. Trousseau sign. *From* Linton AD. Introduction to Medical-Surgical Nursing, 4th Edition, Philadelphia, PA: Elsevier. pgs. 979–1000; with permission.

Maintenance therapy guidelines are not well established. Typical long-term treatment recommendations are with calcium carbonate or calcium citrate and calcitriol with or without cholecalciferol. Calcium dosing is typically 1500 to 9450 mg divided into twice daily or 3 times daily dosing to ensure optimal absorption.[2] Use of calcitriol 0.125 to 4.0 μg daily is recommended to allow for increased calcium absorption in the intestine.[2] In cases of persistent hypocalcemia, additional supplementation with ergocalciferol and/or use of thiazide diuretics can allow for further intestinal calcium absorption and renal calcium reabsorption, respectively.[2]

In 2015, a recombinant human PTH therapy was approved as an adjunct when a patient is poorly controlled on traditional calcium and vitamin D supplementation.[2] Trial information shows that supplementation is decreased by 50%, urinary calcium excretion is decreased, and quality of life is improved.[5] However, there are insufficient data to determine the long-term effects on a decrease in nephrolithiasis and improvement in bone mineralization. Importantly, recombinant human PTH has a Risk Evaluation and Mitigation Strategy program for osteosarcoma found only in the higher doses given to rats.[2]

Misconception 1: The goal in treating hypocalcemia secondary to hypoparathyroidism is obtaining a normal serum calcium level

Contrary to some perceptions, reaching a normal serum calcium level in hypocalcemia secondary to hypoparathyroidism not only is unnecessary for symptomatic relief but also predisposes the patient to dangerous adverse effects. Instead, the therapeutic goal is to use the lowest effective dose of calcium and calcitriol (with or without cholecalciferol and magnesium) in order to achieve symptomatic relief while targeting low-normal or even marginally low serum calcium 8.0 to 9.0 mg/dL[6] with normal 24-hour urine calcium. Targeting normal calcium levels in hypoparathyroidism requires large doses of calcium, and calcitriol and (in the absence of iPTH-induced renal calcium reabsorption) the burden of calcium excretion in the kidneys is increased. Normalization of serum calcium can subsequently cause renal disease secondary to hypercalciuria, including nephrolithiasis, nephrocalcinosis, and renal failure. Therefore, 24-hour urine calcium monitoring in addition to serologic calcium measures is prudent in maintenance therapy of hypocalcemia secondary to hypoparathyroidism.[6]

HYPERCALCEMIA

Elevated serum calcium is most often found incidentally in an asymptomatic patient.[3] Classically, symptoms may include "bones, stones, abdominal groans, and psychic moans," referring to bone pain or pathologic fracture, kidney stones, a constellation of gastrointestinal symptoms, and central nervous system disturbance, including fatigue, lethargy, depression, and memory loss. For those patients that are symptomatic, nephrolithiasis is the most prevalent concern and is followed distantly by documented bone disease and complaints of muscle weakness or pain.[3] Bone disease includes osteopenia, osteoporosis, or pathologic fracture. Patients may also report nonspecific constitutional symptoms of malaise, and mood lability or disturbances (**Box 1**).

Causes of Hypercalcemia

Whether hypercalcemia is found incidentally or on an investigation for concerning symptoms, a thorough review of the patient's medications, supplements, past medical history, family history, and symptoms is essential. Causes vary greatly with PHPT and malignancy, accounting for greater than 90% of cases, with 80% to 85% of PHPT due to single adenoma.[1,7] PHPT must be distinguished from the less common secondary

> **Box 1**
> **Symptoms of hypercalcemia**
>
> Bone mineral density depletion on 3-view DEXA scan (preferential depletion from the distal third of the forearm)
>
> Pathologic fracture
>
> Nephrolithiasis
>
> Myalgias/arthralgias
>
> Muscle weakness
>
> Mood disturbances
>
> Fatigue/lethargy
>
> *Data from* AACE/AAES Task Force on Primary Hyperparathyroidism. The American Association of Clinical Endocrinologists and the American Association of Endocrine Surgeons Position Statement on the diagnosis and management of primary hyperparathyroidisim. Endocr Pract 2005;11(1):49–54.

and tertiary hyperparathyroidism. Secondary hyperparathyroidism is characterized by low normal calcium with compensatory elevated iPTH levels seen in the presence of vitamin D deficiency or in renal insufficiency. Tertiary hyperparathyroidism refers to high PTH levels after longstanding secondary hyperparathyroidism, as seen in chronic kidney disease or refractory hyperparathyroidism after renal transplant (**Table 1**).

Patients consuming excessive amounts of over-the-counter vitamin D supplements or prescription calcitriol (1,25-dihydroxyvitamin D3) allows for increased intestinal calcium absorption.[4] Conditions such as sarcoidosis that cause increased 1,25-dihydroxyvitamin D3 levels will cause a similar effect.[4] Oral dosages of calcium exceeding the renal tubular calcium capacity occur in excessively high calcium supplementation or in chronic kidney disease due to low glomerular filtration rate.[4]

Thiazide diuretics work by inhibiting reabsorption of sodium in the distal convoluted tubule. Lower serum levels of sodium decrease the activity of the sodium/calcium antiporter, resulting in increased calcium retention. Similarly, chronic lithium use can cause hypercalcemia by causing increased calcium reabsorption in the loop of Henle and further increase calcium levels by interfering with the negative feedback mechanism on the parathyroid glands (**Box 2**).[9]

Both endocrine and nonendocrine conditions can cause hypercalcemia as a byproduct of the disease process. Hyperthyroidism primarily increases serum calcium levels through increased osteoclastic bone turnover.[4,7,10] Immobility suppresses osteoblastic activity and somewhat increases osteoclastic activity, promoting bone resorption.[4,7,11] Hypercalcemia may also be present in malignancy due to local osteolysis in multiple

Table 1	
Causes of hyperparathyroidism	
Hyperparathyroidism[8]	**Causes**
Primary	Parathyroid adenoma(s) 85%–90%; parathyroid hyperplasia 10%; parathyroid carcinoma 1%
Secondary	Secondary to vitamin D deficiency or renal insufficiency
Tertiary	Excessive iPTH secretion after longstanding secondary hyperparathyroidism or refractory hyperparathyroidism after renal transplant

---

Box 2
Medication and supplement-induced hypercalcemia

Excess over-the-counter vitamin D supplements (cholecalciferol, ergocalciferol) or prescription calcitriol (1,25-dihydroxyvitamin D3)

Oral dosages of calcium exceeding the renal tubular calcium capacity

Thiazide diuretics

Chronic lithium use

---

myeloma[4,7] or with humoral hypercalcemia from elevated PTH-related protein. Familial hypercalcemic hypocalciuria (FHH) is a benign genetic condition in which the calcium receptor is mutated, resulting in elevated serum calcium levels with or without elevated iPTH levels.[12] FHH usually causes no adverse effect and does not require treatment. Moreover, surgery is ineffective as hypercalcemia will persist even after surgery in patients with FHH. FHH is differentiated from PHPT with low 24-hour urine calcium/creatinine clearance ratio.[4,7,12,13] It is imperative to differentiate FHH from PHPT in order to avoid unnecessary surgery.

Diagnostic Approach

After detecting hypercalcemia, again the first step is to confirm the abnormal finding with assessing serum calcium levels in the context of albumin.[3] Ionized calcium can be helpful to assess a patient with symptoms of hypercalcemia but with normal total serum calcium levels. As previously discussed, most outpatient hypercalcemia cases are caused by PHPT. Therefore, in the absence of concerning examination findings, family history, or past medical history, the evaluation should be targeted as such with evaluation of iPTH and 24-hour urine calcium and creatinine as well as levels that can affect the interpretation of parathyroid levels: 25-hydroxyvitamin D and renal functions.[3,4] In the setting of PHPT, the workup may show elevated serum chloride levels and less commonly elevated creatinine, blood urea nitrogen, and bone fraction of alkaline phosphatase.[1]

However, an investigation into less common causes of hypercalcemia is warranted in suppressed PTH, presence of suspicious findings in the history or on examination, or after a negative hyperparathyroidism workup. Such further evaluation includes thyroid-stimulating hormone (suppressed in hyperthyroidism), angiotensin-converting enzyme (elevated in sarcoidosis), PTH-related protein (elevated in malignancy), and serum/urine protein electrophoresis (M-protein spike in multiple myeloma) (**Table 2**).

Table 2
Differential diagnosis and diagnostic studies of hypercalcemia

Differential Diagnosis: Rare Causes	Diagnostic Study
Sarcoidosis	Elevated angiotensin-converting enzyme, elevated calcitriol
Malignancy	Elevated PTH-related protein
Multiple myeloma	M-protein spike on protein electrophoresis
FHH	Low 24-h urine calcium/creatinine clearance ratio[13]
Hyperthyroidism	Suppressed thyroid-stimulating hormone with or without elevated free thyroxine levels

Misconception 2: Normal intact parathyroid hormone rules out primary hyperparathyroidism

An elevated PTH level in the setting of hypercalcemia is a clear indication of PHPT. In the presence of normal vitamin D levels and renal functions, these findings are consistent with PHPT, most commonly because of a single parathyroid adenoma. Appropriate response to hypercalcemia or high-normal calcium level is PTH suppression. Therefore, a normal PTH level with concomitant hypercalcemia is not physiologic and is considered inappropriate, supporting the diagnosis of PHPT.[1] This diagnosis can be further supported with a finding of high-normal or elevated 24-hour urine to creatinine ratio, which rules out FHH (**Table 3**).

Misconception 3: If imaging does not show a parathyroid adenoma, parathyroidectomy is not recommended

Although localization of a parathyroid adenoma on imaging can help to confirm a diagnosis of PHPT, the absence of an adenoma does not rule out the condition. Instead, parathyroid imaging is useful in preoperative mapping for parathyroidectomy.[1,14] The most commonly used imaging modality is ^{99m}Tc-sestamibi scan accompanied by single-photon emission computed tomography (CT). Adjunct imaging studies include parathyroid ultrasonography, and more recently, 3-dimensional CT scan with added sensitivity.[14] A diagnosis of PHPT is made by evaluating serologic and urine studies as above and can be supported with localization of an adenoma. In cases of suspected PHPT with negative localization, the patient can be referred for

Table 3
Making a diagnosis of primary hyperparathyroidism

Diagnostic Study	Positive Finding	Necessary for Diagnosis?
iPTH	Elevated or normal	Yes
24-h urine calcium and creatinine	Elevated or high-normal	Yes
25-hydroxyvitamin D	Normal	Yes, low vitamin D may indicate secondary hyperparathyroidism and high vitamin D may indicate hypercalcemia due to vitamin D toxicity
Renal functions	Normal	Yes, low renal function may indicate tertiary hyperparathyroidism
Chloride	Elevated	No
Alkaline phosphatase	Elevated	No
Parathyroid US	Localization of adenoma	No
Sestamibi scan	Localization of adenoma	No
Intraoperative PTH testing	Elevated	No, used during exploratory parathyroidectomy after negative localization on preoperative imaging

Data from AACE/AAES Task Force on Primary Hyperparathyroidism. The American Association of Clinical Endocrinologists and the American Association of Endocrine Surgeons position statement on the diagnosis and management of primary hyperparathyroidism. Endocr Pract 2005;11(1):49–54.

exploratory parathyroidectomy, where the diagnosis can be confirmed with intraoperative PTH testing.[14]

Misconception 4: Once primary hyperparathyroidism is confirmed, surgical removal of the adenoma(s) is recommended

The diagnosis of PHPT/parathyroid adenoma alone does not warrant surgical intervention. In select patients, benefits of surgery do not outweigh risks and instead observation alone would be preferred. Intervention with parathyroidectomy versus observation is warranted in the presence of clinical symptoms of hypercalcemia, significant hypercalcemia designated as greater than 1 mg/dL over the upper limit of normal, manifestation of osteoporosis as a complication, hypercalciuria, and evidence of nephrolithiasis or nephrocalcinosis.[1,14] Concomitant chronic kidney disease stage 3 also warrants surgical intervention because of increasing iPTH levels throughout the disease process, resulting in higher incidence of complications.[14] An ideal candidate with acceptable surgical risk is less than 50 years old (**Box 3**). However, it is prudent to include that most recent recommendations urge the consideration for surgical interventions in all confirmed PHPT in patients who do not have contraindications for surgery.[14]

Emergently elevated calcium levels require immediate treatment, which is not covered in this review.

Medical Treatments

For individuals who do not meet surgical criteria, there are insufficient long-term data for medication intervention. No long-term data are available to support the efficacy of treatment with bisphosphonates, estrogen, or selective estrogen receptor modulators to use for bone mineral density preservation.[14] However, the calcimimetic medication cinacalcet shows promise in lowering serum calcium levels without compromising bone mineral density .[14] Cinacalcet functions by increasing the sensitivity in the calcium-detecting parathyroid gland receptor, which in turn decreases PTH secretion. Individuals that do not meet surgical criteria should keep hydrated and should be reassessed every 1 to 2 years with dual-energy X-ray absorptiometry (DEXA) scan, annually with serologic evaluation and regularly with investigation for clinical symptoms of hypercalcemia (**Table 4**).[14]

Box 3
Surgical criteria for single gland versus exploratory parathyroidectomy

Symptomatic hypercalcemia

Serum calcium greater than 1 mg/dL above the upper limit of normal

Osteoporosis

Age less than 50

Creatinine clearance less than 60 mL/min

Hypercalciuria or evidence of nephrolithiasis/nephrocalcinosis

Data from AACE/AAES Task Force on Primary Hyperparathyroidism. The American Association of Clinical Endocrinologists and the American Association of Endocrine Surgeons Position Statement on the diagnosis and management of primary hyperparathyroidism. Endocr Pract 2005;11(1):49–54; and Bilezikian JP, Brandi ML, Eastell R, et al. Guidelines for the management of asymptomatic primary hyperparathyroidism: summary statement from the Fourth International Workshop. J Clin Endocrinol Metab 2014;99:3561–69.

Table 4 Summary of misconceptions	
Misconception	**Fact**
The goal in treating hypocalcemia secondary to hypoparathyroidism is obtaining a normal serum calcium level	Treatment goal is to use the lowest effective dose of calcium and calcitriol to achieve symptom relief while targeting low-normal/marginally low serum calcium 8.0–9.0 mg/dL with normal 24-h urine calcium to prevent renal disease secondary to hypercalciuria
Normal iPTH rules out PHPT	Appropriate PTH response to hypercalcemia/high-normal calcium level is suppression. Therefore, a normal PTH level with concomitant hypercalcemia is not physiologic and is consistent with PHPT
If imaging does not show a parathyroid adenoma, parathyroidectomy is not recommended	The role of parathyroid imaging is in preoperative adenoma localization and is not required in the diagnosis of PHPT
Once PHPT is confirmed, surgical removal of the adenoma(s) is recommended	Patients who meet criteria should be referred for parathyroidectomy: symptomatic hypercalcemia, serum calcium >1 mg/dL above the upper limit of normal, osteoporosis, age <50, hypercalciuria, evidence of nephrolithiasis or nephrocalcinosis, and creatinine clearance <60 cc/min. However, consider surgical intervention in all confirmed primary hyperparathyroidism in the absence of surgical contraindications

CASE STUDIES
Case Study 1

A 38-year-old man presents to the surgery clinic 1 week status post total thyroidectomy for benign multinodular goiter. He notes concerns about malaise as well as tingling in his fingers. Examination and vital signs are within normal limits. What is the most likely diagnosis based on this information?

1. Thyroid malignancy
2. Postoperative hypercalcemia
3. Postoperative hypoparathyroidism
4. Anesthesia reaction
5. Postoperative infection

The correct answer is (3): This patient's symptoms and recent history are concerning for hypocalcemia secondary to hypoparathyroidism. Damage to parathyroid tissue during thyroidectomy can lead to transient versus permanent hypocalcemia. This can result in malaise and hyperesthesias periorally and to the distal extremities.

Patients with thyroid malignancy are frequently asymptomatic, and the diagnosis is unlikely due to recent benign pathology. Hypercalcemia is unlikely after thyroidectomy, and hyperesthesias are inconsistent with this diagnosis. Complaints of myalgias, arthralgias, muscle weakness, mood lability, and fatigue would be more consistent with a finding of hypercalcemia. As this patient is afebrile and does not have concerns about subjective fever, chills, or sweats, infection is unlikely.

After confirming the diagnosis, this patient is started on replacement with calcium and calcitriol. He returns to the clinic for reassessment 1 month later and notes persistent hyperesthesias. Updated serum calcium is 8.3 mg/dL (8.3–10.3 mg/dL). What is the next most appropriate step?

1. Continue the current supplementation regimen because serum calcium levels are now within normal limits.
2. Decrease the current regimen because his symptoms are concerning for relative hypercalcemia.
3. Increase the supplementation because serum calcium is near the lower limit of the normal range.
4. Check 24-hour urine calcium-to-creatinine ratio, and if low or normal, then increase supplementation.

The correct answer is (4): The 3 treatment goals in hypocalcemia secondary to hypoparathyroidism are (a) symptomatic relief, (b) low-normal or marginally low serum calcium 8.0 to 9.0 mg/dL, and (c) maintaining normal 24-hour urine calcium. This patient has met one treatment goal of normal/low-normal serum calcium but remains symptomatic. His 24-hour urine calcium is unknown. In this particular case, continuing the current regimen may be the prudent course of action, but the evaluation is incomplete without 24-hour urine calcium assessment.

Increasing the regimen without assessing the degree of renal burden increases the potential for renal disease secondary to hypercalciuria. Decreasing the regimen is not recommended because this patient remains symptomatic for hypocalcemia and not hypercalcemia.

Case Study 2

A 49-year-old woman presents to the endocrinology clinic for management of a new diagnosis of osteoporosis found on postmenopausal screening DEXA scan 3 months ago with T-score lumbar spine −1.9%, femoral neck −2.8%, and distal forearm −3.2%. She has no previous DEXA scans for comparison. She complains of bilateral hip and knee pain as well as increased mood lability. Last menstrual period was 15 months ago. No other known medical history. There is no concerning family history. She has normal vital signs and no concerning examination findings. This patient's presentation is concerning for the following:

1. Hypoparathyroidism
2. Primary hyperparathyroidism
3. Tertiary hyperparathyroidism
4. Local osteolysis in multiple myeloma
5. Spontaneous bilateral hip fractures

The correct answer is (2): Due to the severity of osteoporosis given this patient's age and duration of menopause, there is a concern for a secondary underlying contributing factor. Moreover, the corresponding symptoms of arthralgias and mood disturbances are concerning for hypercalcemia. The most common cause of hypercalcemia is primary hyperparathyroidism. Hypoparathyroidism does not increase the risk of osteoporosis.

Without any concerning past medical history, tertiary hyperparathyroidism is unlikely. Multiple myeloma is a less common cause of hypercalcemia that should not be suspected initially unless a patient presents with back pain and severe demineralized bone in spine, particularly in a younger patient. Although nontraumatic hip fractures may be present in severe osteoporosis, bilateral fractures are unlikely, and this patient's concomitant mood lability is more concerning for a systemic abnormality.

Laboratory evaluation reveals normal renal functions, serum calcium 10.7 mg/dL (8.3–10.3 mg/dL), corrected calcium 11.1 mg/dL, iPTH 53 pg/mL (14–64 pg/mL), and 24-hour calcium/creatinine ratio 301 mg/g creatinine (30–275 mg/g creatinine). Follow-up sestamibi scan and parathyroid ultrasound (US) are negative for parathyroid adenoma. Are these findings consistent with the suspected diagnosis of primary hyperparathyroidism?

Yes, these data are sufficient to confirm primary hyperparathyroidism. In the setting of hypercalcemia, the appropriate response is iPTH suppression. Therefore, a normal iPTH level is pathologic. Elevated 24-hour urine calcium/creatinine ratio distinguishes this case from familial hypercalcemic hypocalciuria, which is unlikely to cause osteoporosis. Localization of parathyroid adenoma is not required for the diagnosis.

In this patient's case, would surgical intervention or observation be most appropriate?

This patient is symptomatic for hypercalcemia with arthralgias and mood disturbances, and she has documented osteoporosis. Moreover, she is an ideal surgical candidate due to her age less than 50 years old. Therefore, referral for exploratory parathyroidectomy is the most appropriate management.

Case Study 3

A 32-year-old woman presents to the endocrinology clinic for a finding of incidental hypercalcemia on annual examination. She notes a past medical history of right carpal tunnel syndrome due to a 10-year history as a court stenographer. She is otherwise healthy without concerning personal or family history. She denies use of any medications or over-the-counter supplementation. She complains of right wrist pain and otherwise feels well. Review of her medical records shows normal renal functions and serum calcium 10.9 mg/dL (8.3–10.3 mg/dL). Follow-up evaluation in clinic shows: 25-hydroxyvitamin D 62 ng/mL (30–79 ng/mL), iPTH 67 pg/mL (14–64 pg/mL), and 24-hour calcium/creatinine ratio 8 mg/g creatinine (30–275 mg/g creatinine). DEXA scan shows T-score lumbar spine −0.2 and femoral neck 0.3. These findings are most consistent with a diagnosis of

1. Hypercalcemia secondary to vitamin D toxicity
2. Sarcoidosis
3. Primary hyperparathyroidism
4. Secondary hyperparathyroidism
5. Familial hypercalcemic hypocalciuria

The correct answer is (5): Hypercalcemia in the setting of high-normal or high iPTH and low 24-hour urine calcium is consistent with a diagnosis of FHH. Supporting information is normal DEXA scan and absence of concerning symptoms for hypercalcemia. This patient has joint pain that is localized to an area of known carpal tunnel syndrome only. The vitamin D level and renal functions are within normal ranges and iPTH is marginally elevated, ruling out multiple options: sarcoidosis, secondary hyperparathyroidism, and hypercalcemia secondary to vitamin D toxicity. Low 24-hour urine calcium is inconsistent with primary hyperparathyroidism and is essential in distinguishing this case of hypercalcemia as FHH.

What is the most appropriate treatment recommendation for this patient?

No treatment is recommended because FHH is a benign condition not causing manifestations of hypercalcemia. Therefore, there is no role of treatment with parathyroidectomy or cinacalcet in this condition.

SUMMARY

Maintenance of normal serum calcium levels is critical for healthy neurologic and musculoskeletal function. Any variation in calcium levels outside of the normal range must be evaluated in order to correct or treat the underlying cause and restore calcium homeostasis.

Hypocalcemia is often caused by postoperative hypoparathyroidism as a transient or permanent consequence of thyroidectomy. Presentation ranges from asymptomatic to perioral/distal extremity hyperesthesias to muscle tetany. Accurate calcium levels can be ascertained using corrected calcium in the context of albumin levels, or ionized calcium can be assessed when hypocalcemia is suspected despite normal total calcium levels. Treatment is replacement with calcium and calcitriol with or without cholecalciferol and magnesium. Therapeutic goals are correcting hypocalcemia symptoms while maintaining a low or low-normal serum calcium level and normal 24-hour urine calcium excretion. Targeting normal or mid-normal serum calcium can lead to hypercalciuria and associated renal disease, such as nephrocalcinosis, nephrolithiasis, and renal failure.

Patients presenting with hypercalcemia may be asymptomatic or may report fatigue, mood lability, arthralgias, myalgias, or muscle weakness. There may be a history of nephrolithiasis, bone mineral depletion, or pathologic fracture. Most outpatient hypercalcemia is caused by PHPT, or excess PTH secondary to parathyroid adenoma(s). Alternative causes can vary from tertiary hyperparathyroidism, thiazide diuretic or lithium use, excess calcium or vitamin D supplementation, immobility, malignancy, sarcoidosis, or FHH.

PHPT is classically characterized by elevated calcium, iPTH, and 24-hour urine calcium levels. However, a normal iPTH level in the presence of high or high-normal calcium does not rule out PHPT as the physiologic response to hypercalcemia is PTH suppression. Any other finding is pathologic and concerning for PHPT. Moreover, a normal parathyroid US or sestamibi scan does not rule out an adenoma and instead should be used for preoperative mapping. Undertaking the risks associated with surgical resection is warranted in cases with significant hypercalcemia (>1 mg/L above the upper limit of normal range), osteoporosis, significant symptoms of hypercalcemia, or creatinine clearance less than 60 mL/min, and a candidate under 50 years old to minimize the risk of complications. In addition, the most recent recommendations encourage consideration for surgical intervention in patients without contraindication. Alternatively, treatment with the calcimimetic cinacalcet shows promise for patients who are not surgical candidates, but more data are needed to determine the safety and efficacy of long-term treatment with this medication.

REFERENCES

1. AACE/AAES Task Force on Primary Hyperparathyroidism. The American Association of Clinical Endocrinologists and the American Association of Endocrine Surgeons Position Statement on the diagnosis and management of primary hyperparathyroidisim. Endocr Pract 2005;11(1):49–54.
2. Stack BC Jr, Bimston DN, Bodenner DL, et al. American Association of Clinical Endocrinologists and American College of Endocrinology Disease State clinical review: postoperative hypoparathyroidism—definitions and management. Endocr Pract 2015;21(6):674–85.
3. Michels TC, Kelly KM. Parathyroid disorders. Am Fam Physician 2013;88(4): 249–57.

4. Peacock M. Calcium metabolism in health and disease. Clin J Am Soc Nephrol 2010;5:S23–30.

5. Mannstadt M, Clarke BL, Vokes T, et al. Efficacy and safety of recombinant human parathyroid hormone (1-84) in hypoparathyroidism (REPLACE): a double-blind, placebo-controlled, randomized, phase 3 study. Lancet Diabetes Endocrinol 2013;1:275–83.

6. Horwitz MJ, Stewart AF. Hypoparathyroidism: is it time for replacement therapy. J Clin Endocrinol Metab 2008;93(9):3307–9.

7. Carroll MF, Schade DS. A practical approach to hypercalcemia. Am Fam Physician 2003;67(9):1959–66.

8. Kim, Lawrence. Hyperparathyroidism. Medscape. Available at: http://emedicine.medscape.com/article/127351-overview#showall. Accessed July 27, 2015.

9. McHenry CR, Lee K. Lithium therapy and disorders of the parathyroid glands. Endocr Pract 1996;2(2):103–9.

10. Gupta A, Gliden J. Hypercalcemia in a patient with hyperthyroidism. Endocrine Society's 97th Annual Meeting and Expo. Available at: http://press.endocrine.org/doi/abs/10.1210/endo-meetings.2015.THPTA.8.SAT-054#sthash.vElilfQC.dpuf. Accessed July 27, 2015.

11. Lim R, et al. Immobility: a rare cause of hypercalcaemia. Endocr Abstr 2011;25:22.

12. Jeena V, Thereasa R, Camilo J. Benign familial hypocalciuric hypercalcemia. Endocr Pract 2011;17(Suppl 1):13–7.

13. Foley K, Boccuzzi L. Urine calcium: laboratory measurement and clinical utility. Lab Med 2010;41(11):683–6.

14. Bilezikian JP, Brandi ML, Eastell R, et al. Guidelines for the management of asymptomatic primary hyperparathyroidism: summary statement from the Fourth International Workshop. J Clin Endocrinol Metab 2014;99:3561–9.

Printed and bound by CPI Group (UK) Ltd, Croydon, CR0 4YY

07/10/2024

01040505-0010